The Prospective Mother

by J. Morris Slemons

PREFACE

This book, written for women who have no special knowledge of medicine, aims to answer the questions which occur to them in the course of pregnancy. Directions for safeguarding their health have been given in detail, and emphasis has been placed upon such measures as may serve to prevent serious complications. Treatment of such conditions has not been discussed, as it can be judiciously carried out only by a physician who has the opportunity to observe and study the individual patient. Furthermore, if there is to be notable improvement in the management of cases of childbirth, the appearance of untoward symptoms should not be awaited before consulting a physician; on the contrary, prospective mothers must be taught that they should be under competent medical supervision throughout pregnancy.

At present intelligent women demand some knowledge of the anatomical and physiological changes incident to the development of the embryo and the birth of the child. These subjects do not readily lend themselves to popular description, but I have told the story as simply as possible, following in a general way the text-book of my teacher and friend, Professor J. Whitridge Williams; indeed, my main purpose has been to reproduce his book "in words of one syllable." The use of a number of technical words has been unavoidable, and, though their meaning has been given in the context, it has not been feasible to repeat the definition every time an unfamiliar term was used. On that account a glossary has been provided.

It is with pleasure that I avail myself of this opportunity to acknowledge the cheerfully given assistance of many friends. In particular I wish to thank Doctor Henry M. Hurd, until recently Superintendent of the Johns Hopkins Hospital, for his interest and advice. I am also under deep obligation to my friend John C. French, of the English Department of the Johns Hopkins University, for helpful criticism of the manuscript, and to my colleagues, Doctors Rupert Norton and Thomas R. Boggs, for valuable assistance. To many others--doctors, nurses, and patients--I am indebted for numerous suggestions which have been made either consciously or unconsciously.

J. MORRIS SLEMONS.

INTRODUCTION

In all branches of medicine the master word is _prophylaxis_, or prevention, and its benefits are nowhere more strikingly illustrated than in the practice of obstetrics. In former times every woman who gave birth to a child or passed through a miscarriage was exposed to grave danger of infection or child-bed fever; but at present--thanks to the recognition of the bacterial origin of the disease and of its identity with wound infection--this danger can be practically eliminated by the rigid observance of surgical cleanliness and aseptic technique. Physicians have also learned that the most effective method of coping with other serious complications of pregnancy and labor is by preventing their occurrence, or at least by subjecting them to treatment in their earliest stages; for, if they be allowed to go on to full development, the results are little better than in times past. Furthermore, a careful examination some weeks before the expected date of confinement enables us to recognize the existence of abnormal presentations and of disproportion between the size of the mother's pelvis and that of the child's head. Timely recognition of such conditions makes appropriate treatment possible and practically insures a successful outcome; while tardy recognition is frequently followed by disastrous results.

These few examples give some idea of the benefits of prophylaxis in the practice of obstetrics. Prospective mothers should understand not only that there is an advantage in taking such precautions, but that they may be risking their lives, or at least their future well-being, unless they insist upon competent medical attention. It is true, of course, that pregnancy and childbirth are generally normal processes, but they are not always so. Fortunately, most of the abnormalities give timely warning of their occurrence, and in most instances may be relieved by comparatively simple measures; or, if not, they afford indications for treatment which should lead to a happy termination. The recognition of the existence of such conditions, however, is not always easy, and their ideal treatment requires careful training and sometimes the utmost nicety of judgment. Consequently, if prospective mothers wish to be assured of the best care, they should be cautious in the choice of their medical attendant. As the ordinary layman has no means of determining the real qualifications of a physician, the choice should not be made upon the advice of casual acquaintances; but, instead, the family physician should be consulted, who, should he feel unwilling to assume the responsibility of the case, will be able to recommend a thoroughly competent substitute.

From my own experience as a teacher and consultant, I state without hesitation that in no other branch of medicine or surgery are graver emergencies encountered than in certain obstetrical complications whose treatment involves the greatest responsibility and requires the highest order of ability to insure a successful outcome for the mother and her child. For these reasons a physician should be chosen only after mature deliberation, and his services should be esteemed much more highly than is usually the case.

In order that the principles of prevention may receive their fullest application during pregnancy, labor, and the lying-in period, it is also advisable that intelligent women should possess some knowledge of the Reproductive Process in human beings. This information is imparted by Doctor Slemons' book, which I can thoroughly recommend to prospective mothers. The subject matter has been carefully chosen, and the author has wisely refrained from giving advice with regard to treatment which can be satisfactorily directed only after careful study by a physician. At the same time he has given a clear account of the physiology of pregnancy and labor, and has laid down sound rules for the guidance of the patient.

One of the most important facts emphasized by Doctor Slemons is the value of medical supervision for several weeks after the child is born; this precaution contributes greatly toward a rapid and complete convalescence. During the lying-in period the physician should supervise the care of the mother and the child, should insist upon the necessity for maternal nursing, and should keep the mother under observation until perfectly normal conditions are regained. If the latter duty is conscientiously fulfilled many years of invalidism may be saved and thousands of operations rendered unnecessary.

Although there have been notable advances in the science and in the art of obstetrics since the middle of the eighteenth century, a great many fundamental facts must yet be learned. For example, we are almost totally ignorant of the stimulus which causes the mother to fall into labor approximately 280 days after the last normal menstruation.

There are two points which I desire to impress especially upon the readers of this book. Firstly, that the advance of the science of obstetrics, and consequently improvements in its practice, must depend greatly upon the cooperation of intelligent women. They must come to realize that they will secure the best treatment only as they demand the highest standard of excellence from their attendants; and they can aid in securing this for their poorer sisters and their children by interesting themselves in obstetrical charities.

Secondly, they must realize that real progress in the science of obstetrics can be expected to proceed only from well equipped clinics connected with strong universities, and in charge of thoroughly trained and broad-minded men. As yet such institutions scarcely exist in this country. Women who are anxious to promote the welfare of their sex can find no better way of doing so than by bringing this need to the attention of wealthy men interested in philanthropy and education. Furthermore, they should bear in mind that most of our important discoveries would not have been made had animal experimentation not been available, as it is solely by this means that modern surgical and obstetrical technique has been brought to its present degree of perfection; and further progress can scarcely be expected without its aid. They should remember also that whenever they take such a well-known drug as ergot for the control of bleeding, or make use of many other apparently simple measures, they are unconsciously rendering tribute to this type of investigation.

J. WHITRIDGE WILLIAMS.

Johns Hopkins University, September, 1912.

CONTENTS

* * * * *

The Prospective Mother

CHAPTER I

THE SIGNS OF PREGNANCY AND THE DATE OF CONFINEMENT

The Positive Signs--The Probable Signs--The Presumptive Signs: The Cessation of Menstruation; Changes in the Breasts; Morning Sickness; Disturbances in Urination--The Duration of Pregnancy--The Estimation of the Date of Confinement--Prolonged Pregnancy.

Many puzzling questions occur to the woman who is about to become a mother. Most of these questions are reasonable and natural, and should be frankly answered; but a false conventionality has--until recently, at least-- forbidden any open discussion of facts connected with childbirth. The inevitable result has been that, without experience of their own to guide them, prospective mothers have sought advice from older women, whose experience was at best very narrow, and whose views were often biased by tradition. Or, distrusting such sources of information, they have consulted technical medical works which they could not understand. Either of these methods is very likely to result in misinformation and to cause unnecessary anxiety. Yet no one need be alarmed by a plain, accurate account of Nature's plan to provide successive generations of human beings. Some trustworthy knowledge of a process so fundamental should be part of every person's education; it is especially helpful to women who are pregnant because it affords a rational basis for hygienic measures which they should adopt. A popular work, however, no matter how frank and helpful it may be, will not enable one to dispense with professional advice. For the prospective mother no counsel is more important than this: Put yourself at once under the care of a physician.

Insistence on the importance of medical advice should not be taken to imply that pregnancy is to be regarded as other than a normal process. Its dangers are comparatively slight, as we should expect, since the property of all living matter to reproduce its kind is both fundamental and essential; the continuance of living creatures in this world, plants as well as animals, depends upon the Reproductive Process. And yet, natural as it is, pregnancy may be attended by complications. Such complications, though happily rare, are to be guarded against in every case, and that may be most effectually done if patients are taught to remain under competent medical supervision from the time of conception until several weeks after the child is born. This precaution greatly reduces the frequency of annoyances during pregnancy and also assists materially toward conducting a birth to a safe conclusion. Moreover, if this advice is followed, when complications do arise they will be recognized and dealt with promptly; they will not be permitted to grow more serious until, perhaps, they may jeopardize the life of the mother or the child or both.

The initial symptoms of pregnancy are so widely known that in most instances the prospective mother herself makes the diagnosis shortly after conception has taken place; but now and then pregnancy advances for several months unrecognized and is then detected by a physician who has been consulted on account of symptoms which the patient has incorrectly attributed to some other condition. On the other hand, women sometimes suspect that they are pregnant when they are not; and such mistakes occur because certain symptoms which are implicitly trusted by the laity as manifestations of pregnancy are occasionally associated with conditions quite foreign to it. It is clear that one interested in the matter must know not only what the manifestations of pregnancy are and when they appear, but also how far the evidence that they give is reliable.

The signs of pregnancy may be classified, according to their reliability, as presumptive, probable, and positive. The doubtful evidence appears first and the infallible proof last. No one need be surprised, therefore, if, when her suspicion is first aroused, she is unable to decide positively whether she is pregnant. Physicians of broad experience, possessed of facilities for observation which their patients cannot employ, may find it necessary to make more than one examination before they commit themselves to a definite opinion; in some cases, though very rarely, they must wait for two or three months to be able to do this.

THE POSITIVE SIGNS.--The earliest absolutely trustworthy manifestation of pregnancy is the motion of the fetus. The perception by the mother of these movements, which is spoken of as "quickening," generally occurs toward the eighteenth week, if she has been told to watch for them; otherwise they may pass unnoticed until the twentieth week or later. At first the motion, felt in the lower part of the abdomen, is very gentle; it has been variously likened to tapping, or to quivering, or to the fluttering of a bird's wings. As time goes on the movements grow stronger and occur more frequently; they are, however, perceived but rarely throughout the day and seldom interfere with sleep. Occasionally women are annoyed by the sensation and complain that the child is hardly ever quiet. Even these troublesome movements are never a cause for anxiety; but prolonged failure to feel motion after it is once well established should be reported to the doctor.

In the first pregnancy the passage of gas through the intestines may be mistaken for quickening long before the movements of the child are really perceptible; but those who have once experienced quickening will not be deceived. Whenever women who have borne children are in doubt the sensation is almost surely not quickening. Furthermore, in any doubtful case, the motion should be observed by a physician before being accounted a positive sign of pregnancy. This precaution will scarcely delay an absolutely positive diagnosis, since the proper method of examination reveals these movements to the physician almost as early as the patient feels them.

About the time these movements become perceptible another positive sign is available. The physician whose ear has been trained to catch such sounds when he listens over the lower part of the mother's abdomen will hear the fetal heart-beat. Other sounds may be audible there, but the character and the rate of the heart-sounds are distinctive. Since the child's heart beats almost twice as fast as the mother's, under ordinary conditions it is impossible to confuse one with the other. The mother never feels the beating of the child's heart, but occasionally she will mistake for it the throbbing of her own blood vessels.

Ability to hear the fetal heart not only provides a means of confirming the existence of pregnancy in doubtful cases, but also enables the physician to reassure his patient if she fails temporarily to feel the child move. Sometimes the presence of twins is recognized in this way. Toward the end of pregnancy the heart sounds are also of material assistance in determining what position the child has permanently assumed.

There is a third positive sign of pregnancy to which the physician has recourse, but generally it is inapplicable as early as those already mentioned. In the latter months of pregnancy it is possible to outline the child through the mother's abdominal wall. Although this procedure adds little or nothing to our resources for making an early diagnosis, the information it ultimately affords proves one of the greatest aids in the practice of obstetrics.

THE PROBABLE SIGNS.--Obviously, phenomena for which the child is responsible--such as have just been described--supply the most trustworthy evidence of pregnancy; and these phenomena alone are accepted as positive signs. But there are earlier manifestations which intimate very strongly that conception has taken place. Shortly after pregnancy has become established changes begin in the uterus, as physicians call the womb, and soon reach the point where they may be recognized by a simple examination which enables the physician to express an opinion little less than positive. As one result of pregnancy, for example, the supply of blood is increased to all the organs concerned with the reproductive process. Partly on account of this congestion and partly on account of embryonic development, the uterus becomes altered in a number of ways. Although these changes occur regularly in pregnancy, they may also occur when the womb is enlarged from other causes; therefore, if a physician should make the diagnosis of pregnancy whenever they were found, he would make it somewhat too frequently. With a little patience, however, he excludes the chance of being misled; a second examination, approximately four weeks after the first, will generally place the existence of pregnancy beyond question, for under normal conditions the degree of enlargement which takes place in a pregnant womb during a given interval is absolutely characteristic.

THE PRESUMPTIVE SIGNS.--Although women are most often led to suspect that they are pregnant by symptoms which are of such doubtful significance that they must be regarded as merely presumptive evidence, the practical value of these symptoms is attested by the fact that subsequent developments rarely fail to confirm the suspicion. Perhaps they prove misleading once or twice in a hundred cases; the number of mistakes is small, because the diagnosis is commonly made not from only one of these doubtful signs but from a group of them. In order of importance the doubtful or presumptive signs of pregnancy are these: (1) cessation of menstruation, (2) changes in the breasts, (3) morning sickness, (4) disturbances in urination.

The Cessation of Menstruation.--The failure of menstruation to appear when it is expected is nearly always the first symptom of pregnancy to attract attention, and, as a rule, when this happens to healthy women during the child-bearing period--which usually extends from the fifteenth to the forty-fifth year--it may be taken to indicate that conception has occurred. But there are exceptions to this very good rule. Besides pregnancy we are acquainted with several conditions that cause temporary suppression of menstruation; and to understand its significance we must learn something of the menstrual process itself.

Menstruation is a function of the womb and in all probability is brought about through the influence of the ovaries. The bleeding, popularly regarded as the entire menstrual process, is, in fact, indicative of only one of its stages; the others give rise to no symptoms whatever. What the stages in the menstrual process are, what relation they bear to each other, and what the significance of the whole process is, are problems that have been solved with the aid of the microscope. In this way the mucous membrane lining the womb has been studied both at the time of the periods and in the interval between them, and we have learned that it is constantly undergoing changes intended to facilitate the reception and the maintenance of an embryo. Anticipating these duties the mucous membrane receives a more abundant supply of blood; it also increases in thickness and all the structures which enter into its composition become more active. Unless conception takes place these preparations, which represent the most important phase in the menstrual process, are without value; and therefore failure to conceive means that the mucous membrane will return to the same condition as existed before the preparations were begun. The congestion is relieved by rupture of the smallest blood vessels, and there follow other retrogressive steps which completely restore the various structures to their former state. Then there is a pause, though it is not long, until preparatory changes are again initiated, or, as we say, another Menstrual Cycle is begun. Each cycle lasts twenty-eight days, and includes four stages, namely, a stage of preparation, of bleeding, of restoration, and of rest.

Although pregnancy may become established at any time during the interval between the periods of bleeding, it is more likely to be established just before a period is expected or shortly after it has ceased. Furthermore, whenever conception does take place, the preliminary preparations for the reception of the embryo are followed by much more elaborate arrangements for its protection and nutrition. Under these circumstances the hemorrhagic discharge does not appear.

Were there no other condition to bring about the cessation of menstruation, the diagnosis of pregnancy would be greatly simplified. But any one can appreciate the fact that diseases of the womb may interfere with the menstrual process. Menstruation is influenced, also, by the ovaries. As a result of age, for example, the ovaries undergo changes which invariably bring about the permanent cessation of menstruation, called the menopause. This event occurs prematurely if both the ovaries are removed by operation. In view of these facts it is not surprising that sometimes ovarian disorders abolish menstruation. An impoverished state of the blood, or nervous shock and strain, or constitutional debility may also interrupt the regular appearance of the menstrual discharge.

The value of menstrual suppression as an evidence of pregnancy is not, however, to be discounted to the extent that we might expect. This is true because the ailments which lead to confusion are relatively infrequent, and also because they exhibit characteristic symptoms which are foreign to pregnancy. Often these symptoms are obvious to the patient herself; if not to her, they will be obvious to her physician. It is about the doubtful cases, naturally, that a professional opinion is sought, and on that account physicians are perhaps inclined to overestimate the difficulty women have in learning for themselves whether or not they are pregnant. As a matter of fact, it is unusual for a prospective mother to fail to reach a correct decision--a decision for which she relies chiefly upon the suppression of her menstrual periods.

It is doubtful whether menstruation ever continues after conception has taken place. Instances in which the menstrual function is believed to persist are not uncommon, and yet in all probability the discharge regarded as menstrual has a different origin. In most cases it should be interpreted as meaning that there is some danger of miscarriage. Since miscarriage often occurs about the time a menstrual period would ordinarily be expected, there is unusual opportunity for confusing the symptoms. At all events women err much more frequently in suspecting that they are pregnant than in overlooking the condition. Indeed, pregnancy is not likely to be overlooked unless menstruation has been irregular or suppressed for a month or more previous to conception. Thus, in the case of nursing mothers in whom menstruation is already suppressed and who are, moreover, deprived of certain evidence that the breasts give, pregnancy may sometimes advance several months before it is recognized.

The Changes in the Breasts.--Various sensations in the breasts are accepted by women as a reliable sign of pregnancy; thus throbbing, tingling, pricking, or a feeling of fullness will be mentioned by one mother or another as having given her the first intimation that she was pregnant. A few women also find their breasts become tender immediately after they have conceived; this may be so marked that they cannot bear pressure. But unless such symptoms are accompanied by definite, visible changes, they have no value as signs of pregnancy.

About the end of the second month the nipples become larger and more erectile, and deepen in color. The pigmented, circular area of skin which surrounds the nipple, called the areola, also darkens. The shade that the areola assumes will vary according to the complexion of the individual, growing darker in brunettes than in blondes. Ultimately, within this pigmented circle a number of elevated spots appear about the size of a large shot. These spots betray the presence of tiny glands always located there which, on account of the better state of nutrition during pregnancy, grow larger, and generally become visible.

Usually, after two menstrual periods have been missed the breasts increase in size and firmness, and often the veins which run just beneath the skin stand out conspicuously. Before very long it is possible to squeeze from the breasts a fluid which many persons believe to be milk, though it is really colostrum, a substance that resembles milk but very slightly. At first colostrum is a clear, white fluid, but in the later months of pregnancy it becomes yellow and cloudy.

None of the changes in the breasts are absolutely characteristic of pregnancy; even the secretion of colostrum has been noted in association with various other conditions. Furthermore, as a sign of pregnancy the presence of colostrum is totally deprived of value in the case of a woman who has recently nursed an infant, for a small quantity of milk or colostrum often remains in the breasts for months after the infant is weaned. In general, however, women who have not been pregnant before should assume that they have conceived if, after missing a menstrual period, they note the characteristic changes in the breasts.

Morning Sickness.--Soon after conception many women suffer from nausea and vomiting, especially on rising in the morning. "Morning sickness" usually passes off in a few hours, although it may be more persistent. Perhaps this manifestation occurs more frequently in the first than in subsequent pregnancies, but certainly one-half, and probably two-thirds, of all prospective mothers suffer from it. Usually the nausea begins just after a menstrual period has been missed, and ceases about the third month or a little later.

But morning sickness is never counted an indication of pregnancy unless taken in conjunction with other symptoms, for individuals who are not pregnant may also suffer from nausea in the morning. On the other hand, a number of prospective mothers escape morning sickness altogether, and a few experience nausea at other times of day.

Disturbances in Urination.--It is not an uncommon belief that some characteristic change occurs in the urine shortly after conception. But this is not true; at least no change is revealed by any method of analysis known at present. Yet there are symptoms associated with the passage of the urine which appear very promptly and prevail for several weeks. Chief among these is the desire to empty the bladder frequently; some patients also have difficulty in urination, and a few experience discomfort with it. All the bladder symptoms gradually disappear about the fourth month, but become prominent again toward the end of pregnancy.

Since the inclination to empty the bladder more often than usual may be due merely to nervousness or to many other conditions, this symptom taken alone cannot be regarded as a definite sign of pregnancy. Indeed, it is mentioned, not because of its importance, but to point out that it is in no way connected with the kidneys, as patients are sometimes led to believe. It is a direct and natural result of pregnancy. Since the womb enlarges and tilts forward at a more acute angle than formerly, it presses against the bladder, giving the same sensation as when the bladder is distended with urine.

Although the presumptive signs which we have considered by no means exhaust the list, all the others are totally untrustworthy. Each of the more reliable symptoms, as we have seen, must be accepted cautiously; but taken altogether, except in very unusual cases, they may be relied upon. _If, for example, menstruation has previously been regular and then a period is missed, the patient has good reason to suspect she is pregnant; if the next period is also missed and meanwhile the breasts have enlarged, the nipples darkened, and the secretion of colostrum has begun, it is nearly certain that she is pregnant; whether morning sickness and the desire to pass the urine frequently are present is of no importance._ But the most characteristic evidence, we must remember, is not available until the eighteenth or twentieth week; then the signs of pregnancy are unmistakable.

THE DURATION OF PREGNANCY.--After the existence of pregnancy has become assured, perhaps the greatest interest centers about the date upon which the birth may be expected. Even to approach accuracy in this prediction the prospective mother must be familiar with certain facts which she will always observe, but which, unless she appreciates their importance early in pregnancy, she may fail to record or to remember. In a few cases, however, such exceptional information as knowing the date of conception does not lead to an absolutely accurate prediction. But the deviation from the rule will be understood only after we understand the rule itself, which is based upon what we accept as the average duration of human pregnancy, technically called the period of gestation.

In a broad sense, the period of gestation for each variety of mammal is determined by the time required for embryonic development to reach the point where the young may live independently of the mother. This point is reached more quickly with small animals than with large. The mouse, for example, generally brings forth its young in three weeks, whereas the pregnancy of the elephant lasts two years. In human beings, counting from the time of conception to the time of delivery, pregnancy continues approximately 273 days. This number is merely an estimate calculated from hundreds of cases in which there was no question as to the underlying facts. Individual cases vary notably, and indicate that two women may become pregnant on the same day and yet not necessarily be delivered at the same date.

Irregularities in the duration of pregnancy are not limited to man. Thus, while the mean period of gestation in the rabbit is thirty-one days, it may be either shorter or longer by as many as eight days. Similar variations occur in the pregnancies of all animals, and are, moreover, notably greater among larger animals, since for such animals the period of gestation is relatively long. For instance, the accurate observations of veterinarians indicate that the mean period of pregnancy in the cow is 285 days from the time of conception. This fact notwithstanding, a competent observer found that, of 160 cows, 67 were delivered before the 280th day; 68 between the 280th and the 290th day; and 25 after the 290th day. Although nothing unnatural was observed in any instance, the first animal was delivered 67 days before the last, and in 5 instances gestation continued 308 days.

In ancient times it was believed that the duration of pregnancy was of even more uncertain length in man than in the lower animals; but since the eighteenth century thirty-nine weeks have been accepted as the average duration of the human pregnancy when reckoned from the day of conception. As this date is seldom known, it is most convenient to reckon from the first day of the last menstrual period. Estimated in this way its average duration is 280 days. As this period corresponds to ten menstrual cycles, physicians prefer to describe pregnancy as lasting 10 lunar months of four weeks each. This is equivalent to 9 calendar months, in terms of which its duration is popularly stated.

THE ESTIMATION OF THE DATE OF CONFINEMENT.--Since pregnancy is not an absolutely fixed period, we possess no reliable means of predicting the exact day when it will end. The most satisfactory method of prediction consists in counting forward 280 days from the beginning of the last menstruation or, what gives the same result, counting backward eighty-five days from this date. _To make the calculation in the simplest way we count back three months and add seven days_; this addition is made because seven days generally represents the difference between three months and eighty-five days. If the last menstruation, for example, began on October 30th, we count back three months to July 30th and add seven days, which gives August 6th as the probable date of confinement.

A prospective mother should remember that this prediction is no more than approximate. The calculation does not give the exact date of delivery more than four or five times in a hundred cases. It is accurate within a week in half the cases and within two weeks in four-fifths. We also know that delivery is somewhat more likely to occur after the expected date than before it. But perhaps we shall get the clearest idea of the accuracy of the rule, or better still of its inaccuracy, if we imagine twenty patients to have the same predicted date, all of them giving birth to mature infants. The chances are that only one of these patients will be confined upon the day predicted; nine will be confined before and ten after it. In all probability five of those who pass the predicted day will be delivered within a week and four others within the second week, while the twentieth patient will not be delivered until three weeks or more have elapsed.

Such results clearly indicate our inability to make accurate predictions even though pregnancy is normal in every way. Whenever patients pass their expected date uneventfully, if they will bear in mind that the fault lies with the method of prediction and not with the pregnancy, they will often be saved anxiety. Frequently such discrepancies are attributable to a false assumption, for our rule always assumes that the conception took place immediately after a menstrual period. While this is generally true, the number of cases in which it occurs just before the period to be missed is by no means inconsiderable, and in these we should not expect pregnancy to end until two or three weeks after the day predicted by the rule.

Occasionally patients know the precise day upon which conception took place, and prefer to estimate the day of confinement from that rather than from the beginning of the last menstruation. They may do so by counting back thirteen weeks from the day of conception; but this method also is subject to error for, as we have noted, the duration of pregnancy reckoned in this more exact manner is not constant. Such a calculation rarely offers any advantage over that made from the menstrual record.

Another method of estimating the date of confinement is based upon the assumption that fetal movements are first perceived by the mother toward the eighteenth week of pregnancy; and in consequence twenty- two weeks generally elapse between quickening and the day of delivery. Although such a calculation is far from certain in its prediction, there are instances in which no other calculation can be made. A nursing mother, for example, may become pregnant before menstruation has been reestablished. Under these circumstances, obviously, the date of confinement cannot be estimated in the ordinary way, and it is then especially important to know the first day on which the fetal movements were felt. Furthermore, it is helpful to note this date in every case, since it serves, if for nothing more, to confirm the prediction made from the menstrual record. Besides the two methods just described, which are alike in that they require the patient herself to make the necessary observations, there is a third method of estimating how far pregnancy has advanced, by which the physician is enabled to draw his own conclusions. This method is based upon the fact that the womb enlarges from month to month during pregnancy at a constant rate. Up to the end of the third lunar month it cannot be felt through the abdominal wall; but in the course of the fourth month, on account of its size, it must rise into the abdominal cavity. At the beginning of the sixth month the top of the womb is at the level of the navel, and at the ninth reaches the ribs. The diaphragm then prevents the womb from going higher; and two or three weeks before the end of pregnancy it drops several inches, causing a change in the figure which is noticeable to the patient, since her skirts hang somewhat lower than before. From this time on she is more comfortable, because the lungs are not crowded, and there is less interference with breathing.

These alterations in the position of the womb indicate very satisfactorily the month to which pregnancy has advanced, but not the week and much less the day. They do not afford a more accurate means of predicting the date of confinement than does quickening. The evidence gained from the position of the womb, like that afforded by the beginning of quickening, generally confirms the prediction made from the menstrual history; it serves only occasionally to correct it.

PROLONGED PREGNANCY.--Since birth does not occur in many cases until the predicted date has been passed, it will be helpful even at the cost of repetition to sum up what we know in explanation of such unfulfilled predictions. They are to be explained sometimes by uncertainty as to the beginning of pregnancy, as for example by the supposition that conception took place shortly after the last menstrual period, whereas it actually occurred two or three weeks later. In a few instances, however, errors of observation or of calculation will not account for false predictions.

It is generally admitted that second pregnancies average somewhat longer than first pregnancies; one series of statistics indicates that the duration increases slightly with each pregnancy up to the ninth and decreases after that. Pregnancy is protracted more frequently in healthy women than in those who are not, and again more frequently in those who are inactive than in those who work. With twins, contrary to the popular belief, pregnancy is apt to end before, not after, the expected date. The sex of the child, in all probability, has no influence upon the duration of pregnancy.

As we might expect, individuality is also a factor in this problem. Thus, the period of gestation with some women is regularly longer, with others habitually shorter than the accepted average. Until experience has demonstrated their existence, generally, such peculiarities are overlooked. But occasionally they may be detected from knowledge of the interval between the menstrual periods; an unusually long interval between them, for example, would lead us to anticipate a protracted pregnancy.

Any delay after the expected date of birth has arrived taxes the patience of the prospective mother. The fact, however, that more than 280 days have passed since the last menstruation, does not necessarily mean that a patient has gone "over time." Such a question can be decided solely from the weight and length of the child. Judged in this way, comprehensive statistics indicate that once in several hundred cases pregnancy may be fairly called prolonged. Even in these rare instances an examination about the time of the predicted date makes it clear whether pregnancy should be artificially ended or be allowed to proceed to its natural conclusion.

CHAPTER II

THE DEVELOPMENT OF THE OVUM

The Germinal Cells--Fertilization--The First Steps in Development-- The Reaction of the Uterus--The Amniotic Fluid--The Placenta--The Umbilical Cord.

Pregnancy, besides changing the external form of the body, causes sensations--as for example those due to fetal movements--which are so distinctive that they cannot escape notice. These obvious evidences of approaching motherhood naturally lead thoughtful women to wonder about the hidden mechanism of development, a mechanism which, of itself, causes no sensation whatever. It is for this reason, perhaps, that a prospective mother's imagination is so apt to be unusually active, often picturing absurd conditions as responsible for one symptom or another. Those who give free play to the imagination in regard to the formation and progress of the embryo are pretty certain to arrive at erroneous if not grotesque conclusions; for example, they may attribute a protracted pregnancy to the child's having grown fast to the mother, a situation that cannot arise.

Of course it is not essential that a prospective mother should understand what is happening within the womb. And upon those who prefer to be ignorant of the mechanism of development I would not urge another point of view, for not ignorance but the unchallenged acceptance of "half-truths" and of totally incorrect explanations is the chief source of harm. On the other hand, my own experience has taught me that women who wish to know about development should be told the truth. In accord with this is the fact that I never have more satisfactory patients than those who have previously been trained nurses and who, in preparing for that profession, received instruction concerning the reproductive function of human beings.

A description of development, in order to be perfectly clear, must begin with a word about the fundamental structure of the adult body. Everyone knows that the various parts of the body perform different functions; but not everyone, perhaps, realizes that, in spite of their different functions, all the organs of the body are composed of similar structural units, known as cells. Of course, cells are definitely arranged according to the use for which the tissue that they chance to compose may be designed; they have, moreover, distinctive individual peculiarities which can be easily recognized under the microscope; but the essential features of the cells remain the same, wherever they may be located. That is to say, each cell is a minute portion of living matter, or protoplasm, separated from its neighbors by a partition, the cell-membrane; each has its own seat of government, the nucleus, located near its center; and each, to all intents and purposes, leads an individual existence.

THE GERMINAL CELLS.--Many of the cells in the human body are able to produce others of their kind. This they do virtually by growing and splitting in half; cell-division, as this splitting is called, really represents reproduction reduced to the simplest terms. Most cells can do no more than produce units like themselves. The bodies of women contain, however, a type of cell which possesses a far more wonderful power. Provided the requisite conditions for such development are met, these cells are capable of developing into human beings. Each of these remarkable units is called an Ovum, or egg-cell, and represents one variety of the germinal cells. But the other variety, represented by the Spermatozoon and developed only in the male sex, is also required for the production of a human being.

Every ovum originates in the ovaries. These are organs peculiar to women, having the size and shape of large almonds, and placed in the lower part of the abdominal cavity. Though the ovaries are two in number, one alone is sufficient for every requirement of health. It has been estimated that the ovaries together contain at the time of birth about 40,000 ova, distributed equally between them. Since less than 500 ova are required to insure regularity in the menstrual function, it is clear that, if the surgeon finds it necessary to remove one of the ovaries, the other will provide abundantly for menstruation and for the bearing of children. Although every ovum that will be produced as long as a woman lives has already sprung into existence by the time she is born, not a single one ripens for from twelve to fifteen years. The ripening process begins about the time of puberty, and, unless suspended through the occurrence of pregnancy, continues until the menopause. During this period, which is also characterized by the periodical appearance of menstruation, one ovum ripens each month; sometimes, though rarely, several ripen at once, and this tendency is partly responsible for twins.

The human ovum is a tiny structure, measuring about 1/125 of an inch in diameter. With the naked eye it can barely be seen; magnified by the microscope it appears as a little round bag made of a transparent membrane. Briefly described, the ovum is a single cell. That is, it belongs to the simplest class of anatomical structures, and is one of the millions upon millions of units that make up the body. It contains a nucleus surrounded by nutritive material, the yolk. Yet the quantity of yolk is exceedingly small. In this particular the human ovum differs notably from the egg of birds, as it does also in that it lacks a shell. Obviously, a shell would not only be useless to an embryo developing within the body of its parent, but would shut off the nourishment, which, since the ovum contains so little, must necessarily be provided by the mother.

When the ovum has ripened, it becomes detached from the ovary, and enters a fleshy tube about the size of a lead pencil, known as the oviduct. There are two of these tubes, one running from the neighborhood of each ovary; both enter the uterus, but on opposite sides. The ovum travels down the tube which corresponds to the ovary where it originated. The journey is fraught with momentous consequences, for it is during this passage through the oviduct that the fate of the ovum is determined. If it is to develop into a living creature, a great many conditions must sooner or later be fulfilled; but there is one which must be promptly satisfied. Shortly after leaving the ovary the ovum must receive the stimulus to live and grow; otherwise it will quickly wither and die. This vital stimulus can be imparted only by the spermatozoon.

The male germinal cell is like the female cell in the possession of a nucleus; in other respects it is very different. Longer but much narrower than the ovum, the tiny arrow-shaped spermatozoon is particularly distinguished by its active motility, for it has a tail that propels it. The human male cell must travel some distance to reach the point where it can meet a ripe and vigorous ovum; and since the journey is not without danger to its life, Nature has provided that exceedingly large numbers of the male cells shall be deposited in the vagina at the time of the marital relation. In this way, it is made sure that some of them will travel up through the uterus and oviducts, arriving in the neighborhood of the ovaries.

FERTILIZATION.--Convincing observations upon the lower forms of life, especially upon fishes, have shown that when the germinal cells come near to each other, the ovum attracts the spermatozoon. The power of attraction which the ovum exerts may be likened, most simply, to the influence of a magnet upon iron-filings. While there has been no opportunity to observe such attraction between the parent cells of human beings, its existence is not open to doubt. And it is practically certain that these cells meet in the oviduct, even in that portion of it which receives the ovum just as it leaves the ovary. Thither a number of the male cells have traveled by their own activity; several come in contact with the ovum and one, but only one, actually enters it. Almost at the moment when they touch, the two cells unite so intimately that all trace of the spermatozoon is lost. Fertilization of the ovum, as this event is scientifically termed, has as its main purpose the uniting of the nucleus of a male germinal cell with the nucleus of the female germinal cell. This detail has been carefully studied; we know that the nuclei quickly blend into one, and that the particles of living matter contributed by the male animate the female cell with a new and wonderful activity.

In our every-day way of speaking, fertilization means conception; it is the instant in which a living being begins its existence. There is no longer the slightest excuse for confusion regarding the period at which the life of the unborn child begins. Before the significance of fertilization was understood, it was perhaps not unreasonable to believe that life began with quickening or about the time the fetal heart-sounds could be heard. But now we must acknowledge that both these ideas were incorrect. The animation of the ovum at the moment of conception marks the beginning of growth and development which constitutes its right to be considered as a human being.

Individuality, hereditary traits, sex--all these, we may be sure--are unalterably determined from the moment of conception. The germinal cell forms the total contribution of the male parent to pregnancy; therefore no other opportunity for him to influence his progeny presents itself, and the substance which enters the ovum at the time of fertilization must be the basis of inheritance from the father. It is equally true, as we shall see in the next chapter, that the nucleus of the ovum and the nucleus alone transmits maternal qualities. The material which conveys inheritable characters can be seen and has been identified in both germinal cells; from each of them the fertilized ovum derives equal amounts. As the parental nuclei unite, the material which they contain intermingles and establishes a new being; to attain full development, it requires nothing further from the father, and nothing save nourishment from the mother.

THE FIRST STEPS IN DEVELOPMENT.--Although the identity of the spermatozoon is lost at the moment of fertilization, its influence just then begins to be asserted. In the fertilized ovum the dawn of development is shown at first by unusual activity within and later by alterations upon the surface. Before very long the circumference of the cell becomes indented as if a knife had been drawn around it, and shortly two cells appear in place of one. These two cells in turn divide, yielding four cells which grow and divide into eight. In this manner division follows division until a multitude of cells have sprung into existence, all of which cling together in the shape of a ball. Development always proceeds in the same orderly way; evidently it is governed by fixed laws which decree that the mass shall remain for a while in the form of a ball, though the ball, at first solid, soon becomes hollow.

While these changes are taking place the growing ovum is carried down the oviduct a distance of four to six inches and finally comes to rest in the uterus, where it is to dwell during the months necessary to its complete development. The time consumed by this journey cannot be measured accurately; it may be as short as a few hours or as long as several days, but in all probability it is never longer than a week. Although the element of time is uncertain the method of transmission is well understood. Of its own accord the ovum can move after fertilization no better than before; it is never capable of moving itself. The active agent of transportation is the oviduct, which has been fitted for this purpose with millions of short, hair- like structures that project into its interior. These are closely set upon the inner surface of the oviduct; their outer ends are free and continually sway to and fro like a wheat field on a windy day; and by their motion they create a current in the direction in which the ovum should move, namely, toward the uterus. While passing through the oviduct, the ovum has no attachment whatever to the mother, yet development is going on all the time. It is thus made perfectly clear that development is not directed by the parent. This independence of the parent, though it continues to be one of the characteristic features of the development of the ovum, shortly becomes less evident, for communication is set up between the mother and the ovum as soon as it reaches the uterus. Unless we were warned, we might easily misinterpret the significance of this attachment to the parent. It does not permit the mother, for instance, to influence the mind or character which the child will have. The purpose of the attachment is twofold, namely, to anchor the ovum, and to arrange channels by which, on the one hand, nutriment may reach the embryo, and, on the other, its waste products may return to the mother. The mother may influence the nutrition of the fetus; but she cannot determine the kind of brain or liver her child will have; neither for that matter can she alter the development of any portion of the embryo.

After its entrance into the cavity of the uterus prepared to receive and protect it, the mass of cells sinks into the soft, velvety lining of the organ. Here it is entirely surrounded by tissue which belongs to the mother. But just before implantation takes place the architecture of the ovum is modified in such a way as to indicate the trend of its subsequent development. We left it, a hollow ball passing down the oviduct; had we examined the sphere more closely we should have found its wall composed of a single layer of cells. At one spot, however, the wall soon thickens. The thickening is due to a specialized group of cells which gradually grows toward the hollow center of the ball. A little later, if we study the structure as a whole, we find it a small, distended sac, from the inner surface of which hangs a tiny clump of tissue. The clump of cells within and the inclosing sac as well are both requisite to the ultimate object of pregnancy; yet they fulfill very different purposes. The clump within will mold itself into the embryo; the inclosing sac will make possible the continued existence and growth of the embryo by securing and conveying to it nourishment according to its needs. These two structures, which from now on constitute the ovum, can best be considered separately and in the order of their development. We shall therefore first study the sac and in the next chapter the embryo.

For a time after this sac, or ball, as you may choose to think of it, becomes implanted in the uterus, every part of its wall shares in the responsibility of procuring nourishment for the embryo. On this account the wall, or capsule, is for several weeks the most conspicuous part of the ovum. Its position is naturally advantageous, for, since it forms the outermost region of the structure and comes into immediate contact with the tissues of the mother, it has the first opportunity to seize and appropriate nutriment. Consequently, while there is still relatively little development in the embryo, the capsule of the ovum gives evidence of rapid extension; the wall becomes thicker, and the circumference of the sac increases. The significant thing about this growth, however, is the fact that it does not progress evenly. At some points cell-division is more active than at others, with the result that the surface of the ovum speedily loses its smooth, regular outline. Projections from the capsule appear; they increase in number and in length; and by the end of four weeks the ovum, as yet less than an inch in diameter, resembles a miniature chestnut-burr. To make the comparison more accurate, we must imagine such a burr covered with limp threads instead of rigid spines.

These projections, the so-called Villi, push their way into the mucous membrane of the uterus and serve a two-fold purpose. One of their functions is to fix the ovum in its new abode; and, though the attachment is not at first very secure, it becomes stronger in the course of time and is capable of withstanding whatever tendency the activity of daily life may have to loosen it. The other, and equally important, task of the villi, the majority of which dip into the mother's blood, is to transmit substances to and from the embryo.

We have traced thus far the earliest steps in the development of the ovum. One portion, we observed, was promptly set apart for the construction of the future child; this favored portion became inclosed by all the rest of the ovum, which has a more or less spherical form and is technically called the fetal sac. The first duty of the sac is to take root in the womb, and the second, no less vital, is to draw nourishment from the mother. But neither of these functions can be performed without the participation of the uterine mucous membrane, the soil, as it were, in which the ovum is planted. We must now learn how the maternal tissues assume the responsibility placed upon them.

THE REACTION OF THE UTERUS.--The womb, which is small before marriage, is converted by pregnancy into the largest organ of the body. The virginal uterus, shaped somewhat like a pear, and placed with apex downward, is carefully protected within the bony basin between the hips, which is commonly called the Pelvis. The upper and larger part of the organ, known as the body, lies at the bottom of the abdominal cavity; the lower part, the neck, projects into the vagina. The cavity inside the womb communicates above with the two oviducts and terminates below in a canal which runs through the neck and opens into the vagina by an orifice known as the mouth of the womb.

Pregnancy modifies every portion of the womb in one way or another; but the most profound alterations occur in the body, in the cavity of which the ovum has come to rest. During the forty weeks of gestation the organ grows in weight from two ounces to as many pounds; from three inches in length it increases to fifteen inches; and its capacity is multiplied 500 times.

The mucous membrane which lines the cavity of the uterus responds to the stimulus of pregnancy in a characteristic manner and with a single purpose, namely, to promote the development of the ovum. In connection with menstruation we noted that this membrane periodically prepares for the reception of an ovum. And if the expected ovum has been fertilized, its arrival is followed by arrangements for its protection and nutrition which are far more elaborate than the preparations for its reception. Within a few weeks the mucous membrane becomes half an inch thick, that is, about ten times thicker than it was; and all the elements entering into its composition, become unusually active. The blood-vessels are congested; the glands pour out a more elaborate secretion; and certain cells lay up a bountiful store of material to be drawn upon in the formation of the embryo and the building up of the structures that promote its development.

The ovum is as likely to find a resting place at one spot as another upon the surface of the uterine mucous membrane. The whole of that surface has been made ready to receive it; yet the area actually required to imbed the tiny object is extremely small. As the ovum escapes from the oviduct and enters the womb, it is smaller, in all probability, than the head of a pin. For at least a week after its coming, diligent search is necessary to find the site of implantation. Insignificant as it is at first, however, the region of implantation later becomes very prominent, for it undergoes a transformation that the rest of the mucous membrane does not share. That is to say, it becomes the point of attachment of the Placenta, an organ that has the very important function of drawing upon the resources of the mother's blood. As the ovum sinks into this especially prepared bed, the villi are formed. They break open the adjacent capillaries of the mother, thus diverting her blood from its accustomed course. The blood collects in microscopic lakes in contact with the capsule of the ovum, and from them flows back into the mother's veins. Through the veins it returns to her heart, by which it is distributed through the arteries to the various regions of the body. The tiny lakes, in which the villi hang, are thus made a part of the mother's circulation and as such are regularly replenished with purified blood. By this means the ovum receives a rich supply of nutriment, and as a natural consequence its growth is rapid.

Before very long the diameter of the ovum is greater than the depth of the mucous membrane which surrounds it. Consequently that part of the membrane which covers it is pushed into the uterine cavity, as the ground is raised by a sprouting seed. Growth continues, the bulging increases, and extensive alterations are wrought both in the womb and in the capsule of the ovum. One of these alterations will be more easily understood if we still think of the ovum as a seed, for it grows away from its roots just as plants do. Most of the capsule, therefore, is removed step by step farther from its source of nourishment, for the maternal blood-vessels do not follow the expanding sac but retain their original position at its base. Partly on account of the lack of nutriment thus occasioned and partly on account of the distention caused by the contents of the sac, atrophy occurs in the distant portions of the sac's wall. As a final result of these two factors, the maternal tissue which covers the ovum becomes thinned and stretched; it is pushed entirely across the uterine cavity; and by about the twentieth week meets the opposite side of the cavity, to which it becomes adherent. Subsequently, the sac which incloses the embryo becomes everywhere fastened to the inner surface of the uterus and completely fills the uterine cavity.

THE AMNIOTIC FLUID.--The great enlargement of the uterus which is so marked a characteristic of the latter part of pregnancy is due in a measure to the luxuriant blood-supply, for better nutrition always causes growth. In a far larger measure, however, it is due to distention for which the product of conception is responsible. Beside the fetus the inclosing sac also contains a considerable quantity of fluid. This fluid, called "The Waters" by those who have no special knowledge of anatomy, is technically designated as the Amniotic Fluid.

In the earlier months of pregnancy the amniotic fluid is not abundant; later it increases rapidly, so that by the end of the period it measures about a quart, and frequently even more. The slightly yellow amniotic fluid is itself clear, but small particles of dead skin and other material cast off from the surface of the child's body are floating in it, and may cause turbidity. The absence of odor supports the view that this fluid is not the child's urine. The evidence thus far adduced, though not absolutely conclusive, gives good reason to believe that "the waters" are secreted by the inner side of the sac which incloses the fetus. Very early in pregnancy this sac becomes a double-walled structure; and, though its layers are intimately blended, and together measure not more than 1/16 of an inch in thickness, with a little care they can be separated. The outer layer, which comes in contact with the inner surface of the uterus and has to do with the matter of nutrition, is called the Chorionic Membrane; the inner, the so-called Amniotic Membrane, is much the stronger and is devoted to the protection of the embryo, which it completely surrounds with fluid, at the same time retaining the fluid within set bounds.

The amniotic fluid performs many important duties. Perhaps the first, in point of time, is to provide sufficient room for the embryo to grow in. Later, as the fluid increases, it permits the fetus to move freely, and yet renders the movements less noticeable to the mother. Again, the amniotic fluid prevents injuries that might otherwise befall the child in case the mother wears her clothing too tight. Harmful as the practice of tight-lacing during pregnancy is, it does not, thanks to the presence of the amniotic fluid, result in the disfigurement of the child. For the same reason a blow struck upon the abdomen, as in a fall forward, is not so serious as might be thought, since the fluid, not the child, receives the force of the impact. Some physicians believe that the fetus swallows the amniotic fluid and thus secures nourishment. The fluid also serves to keep the fetus warm; or, to be more exact, protects it from sudden changes in the temperature of the mother's environment. Normally the temperature of the fetus is thus kept nearly one degree higher than the temperature of the parent.

Ultimately, the amniotic fluid assists in dilating the mouth of the womb, which remains closed until the beginning of the process that terminates with birth. The uterine contractions at the onset of labor compress the fluid; in turn the fluid attempts to escape but is held in check by the amniotic membrane, which it drives into the canal leading from the uterine cavity to the vagina. Acting like a wedge, the fluid gradually pushes the mouth of the womb wider and wider open, until it is large enough for the child to pass. The sac usually ruptures when that point is reached, the fluid escapes, and in due time the child is born. This is followed within half an hour by the extrusion of a mass of tissue--in reality the collapsed fetal sac-- which in every language, so far as I know, is named the After-Birth. An examination of this tissue at the time of delivery repays the physician, for it is important to ascertain that none of it has been left in the uterus. Our interest at present, however, is to learn how the after-birth has assisted toward the growth of the child.

THE PLACENTA.--The after-birth has puzzled scientists as well as the laity, and not until comparatively recent times have its origin, structure, and use been satisfactorily explained. Its meaning profoundly interested primitive men and stimulated their imagination scarcely less than the mystery of conception. Some uncivilized tribes believed that the after-birth was animated like the child; consequently they spoke of it as "the other half," and often saved it to give to the child in case of sickness. But generally the after-birth was buried with religious ceremony, and was occasionally unearthed later to discover whether the woman would have other children; the prophecy was made according to the manner of disintegration or some other equally absurd circumstance.

The after-birth consists of a round, fleshy cake, the placenta, to which two very essential structures are attached. One of these, running from one surface of the cake, is a rope-like appendage, the umbilical cord, which links the placenta with the fetus. The other, attached to the circular edge of the cake, is a thin veil of tissue, in some part of which a rent will be found. Now, if we lift the margin of the rent, we shall see that the veil and the cake together form a sac which we are holding by the opening. This aperture through which the fetus passed, and it was really made for that purpose, was formerly placed over the mouth of the womb; the sac itself, distended by the fetus and the amniotic fluid, was fastened everywhere to the inner surface of the womb.

It is plain that we have now in our hands the fetal sac, the development of which we have already traced from the beginning. The wall of the sac, it will be recalled, was originally of the same formation throughout; but when the ovum became imbedded in the womb, that part of its capsule which remained in permanent contact with the mother's blood underwent special development, whereas the rest of the capsule gradually pushed away from its primary position and, becoming stunted in its growth, even lost to some degree the development it had attained. This latter portion, the veil that passes from the edge of the placenta, is formed of the two membranes we have mentioned, namely, the chorion and the amnion.

The placenta is, for the most part, a highly developed portion of the chorionic membrane, which became specialized simply because it happened to receive the best supply of blood. At the time of birth the placenta measures nearly an inch in thickness, is as large around as a breakfast-plate, and generally weighs a pound and a quarter, that is, approximately one-sixth of the weight of the child. This relation between the weight of the placenta and of the child is regularly maintained; therefore, the larger the child the larger the placenta associated with it.

The placenta has two surfaces, easily distinguished from each other. The raw maternal surface was formerly attached to the inside of the uterus; the fetal surface, covered by the amniotic membrane, was in contact with the amniotic fluid. Across the fetal surface run a number of blood-vessels containing the child's blood, converging toward a central point at which the umbilical cord is inserted. The point at which the cord is attached affords the simplest means of distinguishing the two surfaces of the placenta.

Our knowledge as to how the exchange of food and excretory products between mother and child is carried on by the placenta has been gained chiefly through the microscope. The oldest medical writings, as we might suppose, express very fanciful ideas regarding the nature of embryonic development and the means by which it is made possible; no rational view of these matters could exist until the circulation of the blood was described by William Harvey in 1628. After this epoch-making revelation, it was accepted as true that the mother's blood entered the unborn child and returned to her own system. But that view eventually became untenable, for it was proved conclusively that there is no communicating channel between the two. For years after that, it was believed that before birth the womb manufactured milk to sustain the child, just as the breasts do afterwards; but this theory also was disproved; and, as I have said, only by the use of the microscope have we learned the truth about fetal nutrition.

When thin slices of the placenta are magnified they are found to contain countless numbers of tiny, finger-like processes; these are the villi, and they constitute the major portion of the organ. The villi seen in a mature placenta are the same as those which projected from the capsule of the young ovum, but not these alone, for many branches have sprouted from the original projections. The primary trunks with all their branches hang from the capsule of the ovum and extract nutriment from the mother's blood which surrounds them, just as the roots of a tree extract it from the soil.

The interchange of material between mother and child as carried on in the placenta can, perhaps, be made clearer if we compare one of the trunks and its branching villi to a human forearm, hand, and fingers. The hand, we will imagine, is held in a basin of water, in which, by turning on a spigot and leaving the outflow unstopped, we have arranged that the water changes constantly. In terms of this illustration, the water corresponds to the mother's blood, rich in oxygen, mineral matter, and all other kinds of essential nutriment; and the fingers are the villi. The blood-vessels in the fingers, to go a step farther, represent the blood-vessels which exist within the villi, connecting with the umbilical cord, and passing by that route to the body of the child. The blood which thus circulates through the villi, it is important to emphasize, is the child's blood; it cannot escape through the coating of the villi, just as our blood cannot escape through the skin of the fingers. Similarly, the mother's blood cannot enter the child; the two circulations are absolutely separate and distinct.

It must be noticed, moreover, that the maternal blood not only brings to the surface of the villi everything the child needs, but it also takes away the waste products of fetal life. Let us select one of the foodstuffs necessary for the unborn child, and follow its course so far as it relates to fetal nutrition. The mother's blood brings sugar, for example, from her intestinal tract to the surface of the villi; through the coating of the villi the sugar passes into the fetal blood, is carried to the fetal heart, and distributed to the various fetal organs. They burn it, deriving heat and energy, and in return give off waste products, namely, carbonic acid gas and water, which are taken up by the fetal blood, borne back to the placenta, and pass again through the coating of the villi into the mother's circulation. These waste products are then transported to the mother's lungs and to her kidneys, and are finally thrown off from her body. Before the child is born, therefore, the placenta, which is an aggregation of villi, acts as its stomach, intestines, lungs, and kidneys.

In every pregnancy the placenta serves in this way as an organ of nutrition, arranging for the passage of food from the mother's blood to the fetal circulation. Occasionally, it is interesting to observe, the placenta performs a very different function, namely, the protection of the unborn child from diseases that may attack the mother. It is able to afford such protection, because the coating of the villi is not permeable to all sorts of substances. In order to pass through their walls, material must be in solution; solid bodies, therefore, are denied admission to the fetal circulation. The most significant result of this restriction is, perhaps, that so long as the coating of the villi remains intact and healthful, bacteria cannot gain access to the unborn child. Since in health there are no bacteria in the mother's blood, this fact has no bearing upon the average pregnancy; but in those exceptional cases in which typhoid fever or some other infectious disease appears during pregnancy, it is gratifying to know that Nature has provided an unusual defense against infection of the unborn child.

That we do not know all about the interchange of substances between mother and child must be admitted; but the essential facts, and they alone are of interest here, have been established beyond contention. There is no doubt whatever that the mother's blood surrounds the placental villi but never enters the child. The fetal blood, on the other hand, is first in the child's body, then in the villi, and then returns to the child again. It never enters the blood-vessels of the mother but passes to and from the placenta as long as pregnancy lasts.

THE UMBILICAL CORD.--This rope-like structure, familiarly known as the navel-string, which connects the placenta and the fetus, is approximately twenty inches long; its length, therefore, is sufficient to permit the newly born child to lie between the mother's knees while the placenta remains attached to the womb. The cord is about the thickness of the thumb and contains three blood-vessels, all filled with fetal blood; in two of them the current is directed toward the placenta, the third carries the blood back to the fetus after it has circulated through the placental villi. In the cord the vessels lie near together and are encased in a jelly-like substance that protects them from injury.

So far as is known; the umbilical cord performs no service other than to link the blood-vessels in the placenta with those in the fetus. Simple as this may seem, it is of paramount importance in maintaining the life of the fetus, for compression of the vessels in the cord would shut off its nutriment. Against such accident, however, perfect provisions have been made; both the amniotic fluid and the jelly-like substance which surrounds the vessels are safeguards which effectually protect the circulation from pressure that might interrupt it.

Frequently, prospective mothers are told they must not "reach up" for fear the cord will become entangled. Such a precaution is quite unnecessary. No matter what the mother does, or does not, the cord will be found around the child's neck at the time of birth in one of every three cases. It is not difficult to understand how this happens. The cord is longer than the uterine cavity and must fall in coils toward the bottom of it. Now, since the fetus is free to move it enters and withdraws from these loops, many times, in the course of pregnancy. Finally, when it takes up a position head downward, as it nearly always does, the head is the part of the fetus which passes through the coil, should one happen to lie in its path. After the head is delivered the physician always feels about the neck to discover whether a loop of cord is there. If it is, he can release it easily. This condition, since it occurs so frequently and since it so rarely produces harmful consequences, should not be considered unnatural.

After the child is born, the physician cuts the cord, and in due time the after-birth is expelled through the same passage as was the child. The expulsion of the after-birth frees the mother of all the tissue derived from the growth of the ovum, for the intricate mechanism that served to nourish and protect the embryo was almost entirely developed from the ovum itself. It is a remarkable provision of Nature that very little of the mother's tissue is cast off at the end of pregnancy; and even this small portion is promptly replaced. By about the sixth week after delivery, the wound which was made by the separation of the fetal sac has completely healed. Meanwhile the mucous membrane that underwent elaborate preparations to receive the ovum, the cavity that was adjusted to its growth, and the muscle fibers that were strengthened to insure its safe entry into the world have all regained their original state. Except for the activity of the breasts, the mother is left in the same physical condition as before she became pregnant.

CHAPTER III

THE EMBRYO

The Development of Form--The Determination of Sex--Twins--The Rate of Growth--The Newborn Infant--Heredity--Maternal Impressions.

The new human being begins existence, as I have shown, as soon as the ovum is fertilized, though at that moment it consists merely of a solitary cell formed by the union of the two parental cells. From a beginning relatively simple the human body develops into the most complex of living structures; and, startling as it may appear to be, it is demonstrably true that every one of the millions of cells which compose an adult has descended from the ovum. Furthermore, the individual himself is not the entire progeny of the ovum; the placenta and the membranes dealt with in the preceding chapter, we saw, were also derived from that same source. They possess only a transitory importance, to be sure, and to most persons they are less interesting than the embryo, yet we gave them consideration before discussing its growth because the manner in which the ovum becomes attached to the womb and draws nutriment from the mother primarily determines the fate of a pregnancy.

Now that we have become familiar with the arrangements for the protection of the embryo, we are prepared to learn how it develops, and may accept the phrase, embryonic development, to cover the whole period of existence within the womb. In a more technical sense, however, the use of the term embryo is limited to the first six weeks of pregnancy and designates the condition of the young creature before it has acquired the form and the organs of the infant; after that time the unborn child is called a fetus. Embryonic development, therefore, in the strictest sense of the term, chiefly involves the shifting of various groups of cells and the bestowal upon them of different kinds of activity. During this period comparatively slight growth takes place. By about the twentieth week, the house, it may be said, is set in order; and there follows a period marked by the rapid growth of the fetus.

THE DEVELOPMENT OF FORM.--A very old explanation of embryonic development was that the process consisted altogether in growth. According to that view the embryo lay curled up in the egg; at the outset it was equipped with organs, limbs, features, and all the other bodily structures found in an adult. In order that the ovum might be transformed into a mature infant, only unfolding and growth were required. After the microscope came into use, however, so simple an explanation could no longer be accepted. Scientists soon realized that the embryo did not exist "ready made" in the ovum, which, even when magnified, failed to bear the faintest likeness to a human being.

Although the microscope made impossible this very simple explanation, it gave in return a truer, if more complex, account of the transformation from egg to offspring. By this means it has been definitely proved that the ovum multiplies rapidly after it has been fertilized, and becomes, as was explained in the preceding chapter, a sac-like structure within which hangs a tiny clump of tissue. This inner mass of cells forms the embryo.

It has proved a difficult task to secure very young human embryos, and many of the ideas we hold relative to the initial stages in the development of man are based upon what has been found true in certain mammals, the class of animals to which we belong. The youngest human ovum known at present has already undergone about two weeks' development, and there the embryo is represented by a flat disk. From this stage to the stage of complete development a satisfactory series of embryos has now been collected, but it is impossible to give here, even in outline, a description of the evolution of the human embryo. No one can understand this intricate subject without the aid of diagrams, models, and other material beyond the reach of all save laboratory workers.

By the end of the second month the development of the embryo has advanced so far that anyone could recognize its human shape. About that time, too, the external sexual organs make their appearance. At first these are quite similar in both sexes; and, if they are used as the criterion, it is possible only toward the end of the third month to say whether the embryo is a male or female.

THE DETERMINATION OF SEX.--The fact that a number of months pass before the sex can be distinguished by an external examination of the fetus has led to the erroneous belief that it can be influenced during the early part of pregnancy or actually determined at will. Various means to accomplish this have been suggested; many of them depend upon modifying the mother's mode of living according as a boy or girl is desired. The most widely known of these doctrines, that of Schenck, was to the effect that the sex of the offspring is always that of the weaker parent. He suggested, therefore, that increasing the vigor of the mother by an appropriate diet would produce a male child, whereas a decrease in her strength would lead to the opposite result. His views, however, were incorrect. After studying extensive statistics Newcomb came to the conclusion that "it is in the highest degree unlikely that there is any way by which a parent can affect the sex of his or her offspring."

Moreover, the results of experimental research clearly indicate that we shall never possess the means by which a mother may control the sex of her child. In the main laboratory investigations have sought to answer two questions. First, at what time is the sex of the offspring determined? and, second, what accounts for the origin of a male in one instance and of a female in another? The study of these problems has been carried on chiefly in connection with insects, worms, and fowl; but as yet insurmountable difficulties have prevented similar investigations in higher animals. For this reason, it is not without the greatest caution that results thus far obtained may be assumed to apply to man.

Sufficient facts, however, have been collected to admit no doubt regarding the answer to the first question. In most animals it is definitely known that the sex of the offspring has been fixed when the male cell enters the female cell, in other words, at the instant the ovum is fertilized. Excellent reasons exist for believing that human beings conform to this rule, and that the sex of the child is unalterably determined at the moment conception occurs. Consequently, any attempt to influence it after that event must prove futile.

For the present, the second question cannot be answered with equal assurance. More than five hundred theories have been offered to explain the relation of sex; nearly all of them have no reasonable foundation and are only of historical interest. The view that girls are derived from the right ovary, boys from the left, has long since been disproven, and deserves mention merely because the laity still believe it. Happily, during the last few years, observations and experiments have been made which greatly advance our knowledge of the subject and give promise of an early solution of the problem. The controlling factor in sex determination has been narrowed down to three possibilities; it is inherited either from the single cell contributed by the father or from the single cell contributed by the mother, or it is determined by the effect these two cells have upon each other at the moment when they unite. In most animal species the weight of authority distinctly favors placing the whole responsibility upon the male cell.

According to recent evidence, there are two kinds of male germinal cells; one kind giving rise to female offspring and the other to male. In all probability, at the time of the marital relation, these varieties are deposited in the vagina in equal numbers; and, moreover, the mode of their production is such as to place absolutely beyond human control the possibility of changing this ratio. Since only one spermatozoon enters the ovum, whether or not the child will be a boy or a girl depends entirely upon which type gains entrance. If this explanation is correct, and it is in accord with careful biological observations, it removes from the mother all responsibility for the sex of her child. Furthermore, since the facts indicate that male-producing and female-producing spermatozoa are present in equal numbers, it follows that practically there is an even chance that an embryo will develop into a boy or a girl.

Birth statistics bear out this conclusion, as data gathered from many countries indicate that when long periods of time are studied 105 boys are born with a surprising regularity for every 100 girls. Thus, the records of Berlin, Germany, for a hundred years show that the maximum difference occurred in 1820, when the males outnumbered the females by 4.79 per cent.; the minimum difference, which was noted in 1835, was .64 per cent. in favor of boys.

No inquiry is more often submitted to the physician by prospective mothers than this, "Can you tell me if my baby will be a boy or a girl?" He cannot. Many rules, to be sure, have been advocated as safe guides toward reaching the correct answer; every midwife possesses her individual formula which she has "never known to fail." But the boastful success depends upon the application of some such method as the following, which I have heard my teacher, Dr. J. Whitridge Williams, expose to his classes. The patient is asked if a boy or girl is desired. She confesses, and is then informed that the sex of her child will be the opposite of her wish. When this guess proves to be correct, there is no doubt of the prophet's wisdom; when it is not, his honor is protected, for the parents have had their hope fulfilled. Their happiness makes them forgetful that the guess was wrong, or, for that matter, that it was ever made.

It was once believed that the sexes might be distinguished before birth by the number of heart beats occurring within a minute. In a general way, the action of this organ in females is somewhat more rapid than in males; and so it was thought that a rate of 144 or more indicated the female and a rate of

124 or less the male sex. But experience has taught that this rule leads to accurate prophecy in no more than half of the cases. As a matter of fact, no means of definitely foretelling the sex of the child has been discovered, and I doubt if it ever can be.

TWINS.--As every one knows, pregnancy commonly terminates with the birth of a single child. Twins appear in approximately only one of ninety pregnancies, while triplets are extremely rare. It is true that even quintuplets may occur, though up to 1904 only 29 authentic instances could be collected from the whole range of medical literature.

Twins are most frequently born to parents whose ancestors have established this tendency; the trait is usually inherited from the mother's family, though occasionally it is passed on through the father. Of course, that does not explain the cause of twins, which in reality may result from either of two circumstances. More commonly their genesis depends upon the ripening of two eggs at about the same time and the fertilization of both by two different spermatozoa. The children, in this instance known as double ovum twins, may be of the same sex or not. On the other hand, single ovum, or identical, twins are always of the same sex; this follows, since but one egg and but one spermatozoon are here concerned. The incident permitting twins to develop from a solitary ovum must occur soon after conception has taken place. It will be remembered that the first step in the development of the fertilized ovum consists in its dividing into two cells. Ordinarily, both these take part in the development of one embryo, but occasionally they separate and give rise to two. Frequently, the presence of twins can be recognized during the latter months of pregnancy, and accurate means are known of determining after they are born to which variety any given pair belongs.

THE RATE OF GROWTH.--When we recall the definite and often marked differences in the physical character of women, such as weight and height, it is surprising to learn that the prenatal development of their children proceeds with uniform speed. One very practical result is that the physician is thus enabled, at the birth of a premature infant, to estimate accurately the period of its development. Various criteria, some of which are easy of application, aid in this determination. For example, the length of the child is practically constant for each of the ten lunar months into which the whole gestation period is divided; if, therefore, the length of the newborn infant is known, the stage of its development can always be inferred. From the fifth month the calculation is especially simple, since the length measured in centimeters divided by the figure 5 gives the month to which pregnancy has advanced. Similarly, we can infer the period of development from the weight, though the calculation is more intricate and the method less reliable, inasmuch as the size of the child in the latter months varies somewhat according to the weight of its mother.

At the end of the fifth month, the weight of the fetus is from nine to ten ounces; whereas an average infant when born at the expiration of the full term of pregnancy, that is, with the completion of the tenth month, weighs about seven pounds. The fetus, therefore, acquires roundly ninety per cent, of its weight during the second half of pregnancy, which clearly indicates that Nature reserves this period of gestation for the fetus to increase in size, a phenomenon less mysterious but no less important than the evolution of the embryo.

Nothing is more valuable than the weight in affording an indication as to whether a prematurely born infant may be reared. It is unusual to raise a child weighing less than four pounds, which corresponds approximately to the end of the eighth lunar month of development (a trifle more than the seventh calendar month). After this time, the prospect of living becomes greater in proportion to the nearness with which the infant has approached maturity. No truth exists in the widespread belief that the seventh-month child is favored above that born later but before the natural end of pregnancy. Experience has taught that the probability of success in rearing the child increases rapidly after the seventh month. This is reasonable on the following somewhat theoretical grounds. The digestive organs later attain a higher state of perfection, and are better prepared to carry on their work satisfactorily. Moreover, the gradual deposition of fat beneath the skin during the last two months of pregnancy materially assists in fitting the child for the conditions met with in the external world, since the fat affords a barrier against the escape of heat generated within the body, making it much easier to keep the child's temperature at the normal point. Even other more technical reasons could be given to demonstrate the error of the superstition regarding the seventh-month child--a conviction endorsed by medical men hundreds of years ago and as yet not discarded by the laity.

When pregnancy has reached "term," the child, having completed its prenatal development, is ready to cope with conditions as they exist in the external world. At term the average child is twenty inches long and weighs 7 1/7 pounds (3,250 grams). The length is remarkably constant; but the weight, as is well known, is often somewhat above or below the average figure. In a general way, smaller children occur in the first than in subsequent pregnancies, and, moreover, may be expected when the mother is a small woman, or poorly nourished, or has worked hard during her pregnancy. On the other hand, a tendency to bear large children is present when the opposite conditions prevail. It is not unusual to see infants weighing eight or nine pounds at birth, but babies of more than ten pounds are rare, and the fabulous, though not infrequent, reports of fifteen and twenty-pound infants are probably not based upon actual weighings, but upon the impression of someone who has merely seen the child or perhaps guessed the weight from lifting it.

Although the fetus frequently changes its position during the earlier months of pregnancy, generally by the beginning of the tenth lunar month it has assumed a permanent posture. It has then reached such a size that it can best be accommodated in the cavity of the uterus if its various parts are folded together so as to give the fetus an ovoid shape. To secure this form its back is arched forward, and its head bent so that its chin touches its chest; its arms are crossed just below the head, its legs raised in front of the abdomen, and its knees doubled up. In this form the fetus occupies the smallest possible space.

With relation to the mother the position of the child, for several weeks before birth, is one in which its long axis is parallel to the long axis of her body. This remains true no matter whether the head or the buttocks are to precede at the time of birth. In ninety-seven out of a hundred cases, however, the head lies lowermost and consequently is the first portion of the child to be born. The opposite position, in which the head is the last portion born, is, even with the most skillful treatment, somewhat more serious for the infant, though not for the mother.

THE NEWBORN INFANT.--The baby at birth is not a miniature man. As compared with an adult its head and abdomen are relatively large, its chest relatively small; its limbs are short in proportion to the body; and at first glance it appears to have no neck at all. The middle point of a baby's length is situated about the level of the navel, whereas in a man the legs alone represent approximately half his height. The changes after birth consist chiefly in growth; but not altogether, since at least one organ, the thymus gland, becomes smaller and completely disappears during childhood, and other organs, especially the liver, are proportionately smaller in the adult than in the infant.

The body of the infant also differs from that of the man in possessing greater softness and flexibility. These qualities depend upon the nature of its skeleton, which is composed of more bones than later in life, when several have fused together to form one to give the mature body a more rigid frame. Furthermore, the individual bones are not so firm, consisting of an elastic material called cartilage, so that some movements which in an adult would cause such serious injuries as fractures and dislocations are perfectly harmless to a newborn child.

The legs are not only short in proportion to the body but are always curved, and the feet are held with the soles directed toward one another, a position clearly abnormal in the adult. But every mother should know that these are natural conditions in the infant, and are the result of the posture of the child before birth. They soon straighten out. The bowed legs of an adult are of an entirely different origin, resulting from a disturbance of nutrition in infancy called rickets.

A small amount of short wooly hair is usually found over the back of a newborn infant. More conspicuous, however, is the presence there of a gray, fatty substance which, though always more abundant over the back, is at times distributed over the whole body; rarely is it entirely absent. The material, technically named the vernix, is the product of the glands in the skin and is a perfectly normal secretion. After its removal, which is readily accomplished by greasing the infant with lard or vaselin before giving the initial bath, it never reappears.

A varying amount of hair covers the head of the infant. No significance should be attached to the quantity, for the conviction that exists, especially among negroes, that a heavy suit of hair for the child occasions "heart-burn" in the mother during pregnancy is without foundation. The color of the hair at birth does not indicate its ultimate shade; changes are often noted during infancy. Similarly the permanent color of the eyes is not assumed until later; at the time of birth the eyes are generally, if not always, blue in color.

A baby's head is a matter of great concern to the family. Occasionally, the skull is round and well shaped from the moment of birth, but more often it is long and narrow; sometimes the form is even startling to the inexperienced. The peculiar shape of the head results, of course, from its passage through the birth-canal and is not a sign of any disease. In a few weeks, or even less, the strange appearance passes away. It is unwise to attempt to alter the shape of the head by bandaging or massaging since the growth of the brain will spontaneously accomplish what is desired; interference can do no good, and may do serious harm.

Nature facilitates an appropriate molding of the head during birth so as to permit its easy passage through the bony pelvic cavity of the mother, and gains that end in two ways. The bones of the head remain pliable until after the infant is born, and, further, their edges are not welded together as in an adult, but are separated from one another by an appreciable distance. During the act of birth the edges are brought into contact or even overlap, materially reducing the size of the head. Within a few hours after birth the bones again spread apart, and some months elapse before they begin to unite; the union is not completed until some time during the second year of infancy.

Many mothers are anxious to know how far the senses of the infant have developed when it enters the world. This problem has stimulated some scientific investigation, though hardly so much as its interest would justify. Two lines of inquiry have been pursued toward its solution. The objective point of one of these has been to determine how nearly the sense organs of the newborn correspond anatomically to those of an adult; that is how perfectly has their organization been completed. The other has been to learn how the infant reacts when the various senses are stimulated; the interpretation of these reactions is, however, particularly liable to error and sometimes amounts only to guesswork.

The organization of the nerves and muscles in the eye is far from perfect at the time of birth. The muscles act irregularly; indeed, the lack of muscular adjustment is such that movements of the eye likely to alarm the parents are regularly observed in very young infants. Furthermore they cannot focus images which fall upon their eyes. The retina, which receives visual impressions, has reached such development at birth, however, that sensations of light can be perceived. For example, if a lamp is suddenly flashed before the face of a newly born baby it cries. From this and similar evidence, indicating that strong light irritates the delicate structures of the eye, we have learned that a nursery should not be illuminated, during the day or night, so brightly as the rooms adults occupy. Certainly several weeks, and probably several months, pass before an infant can see anything save as blurs of light and darkness. Objects, such as a hand, probably appear as shadows, which are not correctly interpreted until late in infancy.

In regard to color vision we have as yet no reliable information concerning children under two years of age. Infants of less than a year have been known to distinguish certain colored papers. But such discrimination is probably due to a difference in brightness of the colors.

Although the organ of hearing is well developed at birth, the drum of the ear in very young infants cannot transmit sounds, as in the adult. For the latter kind of transmission it is necessary that the pressure on both sides of the drum-membrane should be equal, and this is arranged by the admission of air to the middle ear through a passage from the throat. At the time of birth, on account of the swollen condition of the mucous membrane which lines this passage, it is blocked, and the middle ear is filled with fluid; these conditions interfere with the transmission of sound, and consequently its perception is dulled. But even in the absence of a drum-membrane an adult can hear; the vibrations in such cases are transmitted through the bones of the skull, and this very likely also occurs in newly born infants. In most instances, at least, they react to a disagreeable noise within the first twenty-four hours, and their sensitiveness in this direction explains why the nursery should be kept quiet.

Investigators have not come to uniform conclusions concerning the sense of smell and of taste. In all likelihood, smell is not acute at the time of birth. Taste probably is better perceived, yet some newborn babies are said to suck a two per cent solution of quinin as eagerly as milk, though stronger solutions are distasteful. According to the best available information a young infant can detect the difference between a sweet, bitter, sour, or salty taste only when the tests are made with a solution possessing the quality in question to a marked degree. It is common knowledge that babies cheerfully suck the most tasteless objects, and it is not improbable that at first the reaction depends upon the temperature of the object and the feeling it creates in the mouth.

The moment it is born, a baby perceives pressure if its skin is touched. To this sensation, however, some parts of the body are much more sensitive than others; the tongue and lips are most sensitive of all. Heat and cold are probably perceived more acutely by infants than by adults; to pain, on the other hand, babies are less sensitive. An infant is aware of the movements of its own muscles, and also appreciates a change from one position to another, as experienced nurses know very well, and on that account carefully avoid keeping a baby on one side continuously.

The vast majority of movements performed by young infants are reflex acts, that is, the cerebrum, the part of the brain with which thinking is done, is not concerned with their performance. Of these reflexes the most notable are sucking and swallowing, but sneezing, coughing, choking, and hiccoughing may also be observed; stretching and yawning have been recorded in several instances, even during the first days of infant life. None of these movements, we must remember, are produced consciously; the baby cannot reason and does not recognize anyone, even its mother.

HEREDITY.--The transmission of bodily resemblance and of traits of character from parent to child is a broad and complicated subject, whose fundamental principles biologists are just beginning to grasp. The facts thus far established regarding heredity relate chiefly to plants and to the lower animals. There is no doubt whatever that the meager knowledge we possess of heredity in man will be amplified and will ultimately indicate on the one hand the marriages which are advisable and, on the other hand, those which are not. Indeed, the foundations for a science called Eugenics, which purposes to improve the human race in this way, have already been laid. It is barely a decade, however, since our knowledge of heredity has approached that order and system which entitle it to be ranked as a science; and in this brief period great strides could hardly be expected in its most intricate field, that of human inheritance.

The modern teachings of heredity are of interest to us, nevertheless, since they intimate the time when a child's inheritance is fixed and the means by which hereditary characters are conveyed. To understand these fundamental points we must recall that at the moment of conception a male germinal cell combines with a female cell, and that this act, which is named fertilization, brings together vital elements from the two parents. We have seen that the spermatozoon represents the solitary contribution of the father toward the development of the child, and the spermatozoon, therefore, must convey the material basis of paternal inheritance. Similarly we might expect the ovum to be the bearer of the maternal qualities inherited by the child. This is actually true; but much of the evidence is of a technical character and must be omitted. Yet an experiment successfully conducted by Castle and Phillips will indicate, even to those who have no special knowledge of the mechanism of heredity, the important role the ovum plays. These investigators removed the ovaries from an albino guinea-pig, and in their place substituted the ovaries of a black guinea-pig. "From numerous experiments it may be emphatically stated that normal albinos mated together produce only albinos." But in this experiment the result was otherwise, for the albino into which the ovaries of a black guinea-pig were grafted produced only black offspring. The color-coat of her young, therefore, was not influenced by her own white hair, but was determined by the eggs really belonging to the black animal from which the ovaries were taken; in no other way can the result be interpreted. It is certain, moreover, that the mode of transmission of material qualities here exemplified is not exceptional; on the contrary there is no doubt that the ovum always conveys the sum total of the qualities the offspring inherits from the mother.

The germinal cells then contain the material basis of inheritance, and in all probability the substance is located within the nucleus of the cells. This substance had been seen and studied long before its relation to the problem of heredity was suspected. Because it takes a deeper stain than the rest of the nucleus, it stands out prominently when the cell is treated with certain dyes, and this property accounts for its name--chromatin. Under such conditions as prevail just before a cell divides, the chromatic substance is broken up and reassembled in the form of rods called chromosomes. Curiously enough the number of rods is uniform for each species of animal, though different numbers are characteristic of different species; the characteristic number for man is twenty-four.

Unless some arrangement was made to prevent it, the act of fertilization would cause the number of chromosomes in the fertilized ovum to be double the number characteristic of the species. In man, for example, the addition of twenty-four chromosomes from the spermatozoon to an ovum that already contained twenty-four chromosomes of its own would mean that after fertilization the ovum contained forty-eight. Such a result is prevented through the process to which we have referred in the preceding chapter as the ripening of the ovum, and also through a similar process in the case of the spermatozoon. These two processes lead to a reduction in the number of chromosomes, so that finally every human germinal cell contains twelve, and therefore when the ovum is fertilized the characteristic number twenty-four is restored. While we know nothing of the forces which determine, on the one hand, what elements shall be discarded by the germinal cells and, on the other hand, what elements shall remain, it is definitely proved that a selective process always takes place. This fact admirably explains the variation in the characteristics inherited by children of the same family. So far as is known, the traits which will be passed on from either parent are a matter of chance. Whatever these hereditary traits happen to be, the best evidence we have indicates that the problem of a child's inheritance is settled once for all the moment conception takes place.

MATERNAL IMPRESSIONS.--Contrary to all that we know of heredity, the conviction prevails among the laity that the character of a child depends greatly upon the mother's surroundings during pregnancy: this is the doctrine of maternal impressions. As is usual with superstitions, this one emphasizes the unfavorable possibilities and holds that the unborn child may be affected by the mother's unhappy thoughts or maimed by her mental distress if she is exposed to unpleasant sights. For this belief there is no foundation; the cases often cited in its support may be fully explained on the grounds of coincidence.

With the possible exception of such individuals as are spending their lives in solitary confinement, there is scarcely a human being who has not in the course of nine consecutive months some untoward physical or mental experience which engraves itself upon the memory. Prospective mothers are not apt to be exempt from a rule so general in its application, but if by good chance one happens so to be she will hardly fail to hear of the misfortune of others, which, according to the doctrine of maternal impressions, may be equally effective in interfering with the proper development of the child. We should then rightly expect most, if not all, babies to be "marked"-- clearly a situation which does not prevail.

In order to learn how frequently prospective mothers may have disagreeable experiences which they fear will affect the formation of the child, I have lately asked the patients whom I have attended, "Was there any incident during your pregnancy to which you could have attributed the infant's condition, had it been marked?" The babies of all those to whom the question was submitted were normal; yet without exception those whose pregnancies just completed were their first answered in the affirmative. It is also pertinent that one of these patients had lost her brother by a violent and accidental death when she was four months pregnant; a similar bereavement was suffered by another at the eighth month; each was, however, delivered of a perfectly healthy child. Among those with whom the recently ended pregnancy was not the first I found some who could remember incidents popularly believed to have an influence over the development of the embryo; most of them, however, had given the matter so little thought that they could not definitely recall whether such incidents had occurred or not. From a similar series of observations covering two thousand cases, William Hunter came to the conclusion, nearly two hundred years ago, that there was no support for the belief in maternal impressions.

Whenever a child does happen to develop abnormally, it must be clear that, from the very nature of our existence, some incident can be recalled which will satisfactorily, yet unjustly, bear the blame. It may be confidently said, however, that, for every mother whose fears are realized, hundreds are agreeably disappointed in finding their babies perfectly normal. In the face of so many negative instances it is amazing that any person, even though ignorant of medical teaching, should be inclined to attribute abnormal development to something the mother has seen or heard, thought or dreamt, or otherwise experienced while she was pregnant. Yet unfortunately many do believe this. It is worth while, therefore, to supply further evidence, and thus escape any suspicion of unfairness in argument, to prove that maternal impressions are unable to affect the formation of the embryo.

It is found, as a matter of experience, that the superstition regarding maternal impressions generally begins to cause anxiety during the second half of pregnancy; and then such an influence is entirely out of the question. By the end of the second month the form of the embryo has been definitely determined, and subsequently cannot be altered. It is even true that errors in development are most apt to occur within the two or three weeks that immediately follow conception, and therefore occur at a time when pregnancy is not often clearly recognized. Thus it happens that women begin to worry about the influence their minds will have upon the formation of the child long after its form has been established.

Incidents in the life of a prospective mother are in point of fact equally inert so far as their influence upon development is concerned, no matter whether they occur during the earlier or later part of pregnancy. There is never any anatomical means by which maternal impressions could be conveyed to the embryo. Such an influence would have to be exerted through the placenta; and that is impossible. There are no nerves in the placenta to carry impulses from the mother to the child. Even the blood streams of the two beings are kept apart; and though it is unheard of that the blood should carry nerve impulses, if that happened to be the case, it could not prove effective here, for the blood of the mother does not enter the child. It is nourished by food which passes from the mother's blood, to be sure, but there is no more reason to expect this nutriment to exert an hereditary influence than there is to expect an infant to grow to resemble the cow with the milk of which it is fed. With these two possibilities eliminated, no path can be imagined by which impulses might travel from the mother to the embryo.

Scientific investigation has brought to light these facts, as it has also taught the real causation of the disfigurement once attributed to the mother's mind. Departures from the usual form of the body occur during the earliest days of pregnancy and arise in consequence of some irregularity in the process which molds the body-form from a simple spherical mass of cells. Why irregularities sometimes occur is not altogether clear; except in so far as it has been determined that the fault lies within the embryo itself. Whenever these defects are associated with events which have disturbed the mother's mind, it cannot be other than a simple coincidence.

CHAPTER IV

THE FOOD REQUIREMENTS DURING PREGNANCY

The Food-stuffs: Water; Mineral Material; Protein; Carbohydrate; Fat-- What We Do to Our Food--How Much Food Is Needed During Pregnancy?-- The Importance of Liquid Nourishment--The Choice of Food--Cravings-- The Relation Between the Mother's Diet and the Size of the Child.

There is a gain in weight during pregnancy amounting finally to about thirty pounds; exceptionally, it is as little as ten or fifteen pounds, and, at the other extreme, as much as forty or fifty. With individuals inclined to be stout the increase is greater, and it is relatively greater in later pregnancies than in the first. During the early months of pregnancy the weight generally remains stationary or suffers a slight loss; even in those rare instances in which the weight begins to increase shortly after conception the gain is less marked in the earlier months than later. For the last three months the average monthly gain has been found to be between three and a half and five and a half pounds.

The weight gained during pregnancy is not, as can be readily understood, permanently retained. At the time of birth, in consequence of the expulsion of the child, the after-birth, the amniotic fluid, and a varying amount of blood, there is necessarily a loss of from ten to fifteen pounds. Later, as the maternal tissues, whose growth has been stimulated during pregnancy, return to their original condition, a further loss in weight takes place. It is not unusual, however, for women to remain permanently better nourished than before they became pregnant. Under ordinary conditions the food of the prospective mother provides not only for her own wants but also for those of the embryo. Between the two organisms there exists a relation which resembles that existing between a house in course of construction and the contractor who supplies the building material. The mother furnishes what is needed to construct the "living edifice," as Huxley called the growing embryo, but she is not responsible for the lines of the building. The embryo is both architect and mechanic, designing the structure and arranging the "organic bricks" in their proper places. The work of construction necessitates the expenditure of an appreciable amount of energy and the creation of waste products that must be removed, lest they accumulate and interfere with the growing structure. These waste products leave the embryo by way of the umbilical cord and the placenta and return thus into the mother's circulation; ultimately they leave the mother through the same channels that carry off her own waste. First and last, then, the nutrition of the mother and of the child are so bound together that it has been impossible to study them separately. Our knowledge of food requirements during pregnancy has been obtained by measuring the food requirements of the mother alone; and as nutrition during gestation is fundamentally the same as nutrition at other times, it is necessary for us first to consider in general the food needed by the human body.

THE FOOD-STUFFS.--The waste products we throw off indicate that the substances which compose our bodies are being constantly broken down and reduced to a condition such that they are useless to us. In normal persons hunger signifies that they need material to replace what has been used up. The substances thus required, if the wants of the body are to be satisfied correctly, are called the food-stuffs; and they are the same during pregnancy as at other times. The foodstuffs are usually classified according to their chemical properties; on this basis they are placed in five groups: (1) Water, (2) Mineral Materials, (3) Proteins, (4) Carbohydrates, (5) Fats.

In view of the different purposes which the foodstuffs serve, it is convenient to group them in another way. Thus, the carbohydrates and the fats may be placed together because they are the body fuel; their value consists in the heat and energy which they yield when acted upon in the tissues. Water and mineral matter, on the other hand, are never a source of energy; they assist in building new tissue or in repairing tissue that already exists. The proteins are unique, in that they may serve either purpose. Primarily the proteins are tissue-builders, but in the absence of sufficient fat or carbohydrate the body burns protein to secure heat and energy.

Each food-stuff, therefore, serves a distinct purpose, and some of them render services which the others cannot perform. A man will die if either water or mineral matter or protein is completely withdrawn from his diet. Fat or carbohydrate, on the other hand, or even both of them, may be excluded for some time without causing serious inconvenience. It is true, nevertheless, that each food-stuff performs some task better than any of the others can perform it, and for that reason all of them should be included in the diet of an healthy individual.

Some of the food-stuffs, such as water and table salt, come to the body separate from the others; but generally the different types reach us intimately mingled in the various articles of food in common use. Foods vary greatly, however, in the amount of the different food-stuffs they contain. The meats, for example, have a relatively large protein content; in the vegetables starch, which is one of the carbohydrates, predominates. As to the choice of food and the amount that is necessary for the average person, generally the appetite is a safe guide; but the accurate observations of physiologists have gone so far as to determine the exact requirements of the body. Not the least important principle taught by these investigations is to avoid dietary fads, for in arranging a satisfactory diet the problem to be solved is not, What is it possible to live on? but, What serves best as nourishment? The experience of countless generations has taught us that we thrive best on a diet which includes all five food-stuffs.

Water constitutes nearly two-thirds of the weight of the body. As water is constantly being given up in the life process, health demands an abundant supply of liquids to replace the waste. The average daily loss has been found to be between two and three quarts. Of this amount the urine constitutes nearly two-thirds; and the remaining third is eliminated through the skin, the lungs, and the bowels. Although the deficiency thus created is met in part by the water in our solid food, the greater part of the loss is made up by the liquids we drink, and we are warned, in a measure, by the sensation of thirst that they are needed.

Mineral material is of the greatest importance as a constituent of our food. It contributes to the welfare of the body in at least three ways; (1) it gives rigidity to the bones, (2) it supplies an essential ingredient of the living substance in all the tissues, (3) it is present in the blood and in the other body fluids, where it is of service in such vital processes as the beating of the heart, the transportation of oxygen to every portion of the body, and the maintenance of an acid or alkaline condition of the digestive juices according as the one or the other is necessary for the assimilation of the food.

An animal deprived of mineral food will die as surely as one deprived of water. In arranging our diets, however, we are not compelled to take the minerals into account, for, with the exception of table salt (sodium chlorid), the meat and vegetables that we eat provide the mineral material the body requires. Iron, for example, which imparts to the blood one of its most essential qualities, occurs in relatively large amounts in apples, spinach, lettuce, potatoes, peas, carrots, and meats. Only now and then does it become advisable to add iron deliberately to the diet. Similarly lime (calcium) the material that makes the bones hard, is present in quantities ample for the needs of the body in the bread, milk, eggs and vegetables that we eat. The remaining mineral constituents of the body, among which the most conspicuous are magnesium, potassium, sulphur, and phosphorus, occur in foods which we are naturally inclined to take, so that we secure an abundance of them unconsciously.

Protein, the third food-stuff which we must eat to keep alive, contains the chemical element nitrogen in such form that it can be incorporated in our tissues. Although most persons derive their protein in part from meat, milk, and eggs, it is possible to satisfy the requirements of the body on a purely vegetarian diet. Experience has shown, however, that it is both natural and advantageous that we employ a mixed diet.

The property of protein to build living tissue and replace tissue waste probably depends upon several factors; but certainly one of them is the presence of nitrogen. So intimately associated are the consumption of the tissue substance and the elimination of nitrogen that we have no better way of judging the amount of tissue substance used in the body than by determining the quantity of nitrogen that appears in its various waste products. From such investigations it has been found that the quantity of protein required to repair the breaking down of the tissues is not great. The average man consumes approximately a quarter of a pound (100 to 120 grams) of protein daily; but this quantity is in excess of his real needs. Indeed, Chittenden has shown that for various classes of individuals, namely, students, athletes and soldiers, half as much is sufficient. Other physiologists, though admitting that this is true, contend that it is inadvisable to regulate one's diet on such a slender basis. Very good reasons are assigned for the view that more protein is needed than just enough to counterbalance the tissue waste. Thus, in the case of animals, it has been found that a diet low in protein finally causes digestive disturbances and other ailments.

Although it does not seem advisable to practise rigid economy in arranging the protein content of the diet, it is equally important that we should not go to the other extreme. The consumption of over- large quantities of protein, as would be the case if we lived exclusively upon meat, increases putrefaction in the intestines and throws unnecessary work upon the kidneys, which are the organs chiefly concerned in getting rid of the waste products of protein.

Carbohydrate is the name given the group of foodstuffs to which the sugars belong. The food value of cane sugar, the most familiar member of the group, was recognized even in prehistoric days by the natives of India. By boiling the plant we call sugar-cane they obtained a substance to which they gave the name Sakkara, and from this our word sugar evidently originated. The roots of this plant were carried into Europe and cultivated during the Middle Ages. Obviously, its value was and is appreciated, since the cultivation of the sugar-cane and the sugar-beet has become the foundation of a great modern industry.

There are some persons, perhaps, who do not realize that beside cane sugar many kinds of carbohydrate occur in our food. Glucose or grape sugar, for example, occurs not only in the fruit indicated by its name, but also in other fruits, in corn, in onions, and in the common vegetables. Glucose is especially suited to act as nourishing food. In keeping with that fact our digestive juices convert most of the sugars we eat, if not all of them, into glucose, which is regularly present in our blood. It is unnecessary to enumerate all or even the more important compounds included in the carbohydrate group; but everyone should know that starch is its chief member, and that after being thoroughly digested starch enters the body as glucose and therefore serves the same purpose as sugar.

The value of carbohydrates as a source of heat and energy may be accurately measured, and is technically expressed in terms of a unit, called the calorie. As the energy which our bodies require may be estimated in the same terms, it is possible to determine whether or not our food is equal to our wants. Very naturally the energy requirements of any individual are influenced by his weight and by the work he does. But we may take as a standard the results of an extensive study of American families which indicate that women require four-fifths as much energy-yielding food as men. It also seems safe to conclude that a woman weighing 130 pounds who does her own housework requires food every day having an energy-value of 2,500 calories; smaller women and those who do no work require somewhat less. In a mixed diet the chief source of this energy--and the source from which it is most economically obtained--is the carbohydrates.

Fat yields more energy and heat than does carbohydrate, bulk for bulk; but fat is burned by our tissues less readily. We instinctively avoid eating a great deal of this food-stuff; in the course of a day the average person consumes no more than one or two ounces. The natural aversion which many feel toward fat may possibly depend upon the difficulty with which they assimilate it. In colder climates, however, we know fat to be a staple article of diet; and it is not unlikely that the very conditions which make it necessary there explain the unusual tolerance for it.

Fat is more than fuel. Deposited in our bodies, beneath the skin for example, it prevents the escape of heat that we generate and protects us against the penetration of cold. This food-stuff, therefore, contributes in several ways toward maintaining the temperature of the body at a constant level.

Our source of fat is chiefly animal food and in a smaller measure vegetables; but the fat our food contains is not altogether responsible for the fat in our bodies. Carbohydrates, if in excess of momentary needs, are partly converted into fat and stored as such. A reserve supply of nourishment is thus provided, and is drawn upon only when the food that we consume does not contain as much energy as we expend.

WHAT WE DO TO OUR FOOD.--With the exception of water and mineral substances, the food-stuffs must undergo chemical alterations before they are capable of being absorbed into the body; this is the work of digestion. The digestive processes, the main purpose of which is to break up the carbohydrates, proteins, and fats into substances of much simpler chemical structure, begin in the mouth and are not completed until some time after the food has entered the intestine. As the food moves through the alimentary canal, it is mixed with the various digestive juices containing ferments, such as pepsin, which are the active agents of digestion. Although digestive processes go on automatically, they are, in a degree that is far from negligible, influenced by the mind. Thus, cheerfulness promotes digestion, and not infrequently mental depression may be the direct cause of indigestion. Indeed, it is chiefly in regard to the state of the mind of the prospective mother that the existence of pregnancy may be said to have a bearing, whether favorable or unfavorable, upon her digestion.

The digestive juices are prepared in glands which lie either within the lining of the alimentary canal or adjacent to it. In the latter event the glands are connected with the canal by means of tubes. These glands must be warned when to pour out their secretion, and their very first warning usually comes from the agreeable sensations experienced when we see, smell, or taste inviting food. If we are hungry, our viands attractive, and our surroundings congenial, the stimulus excites a plentiful secretion of the digestive juices; conversely, the opposite conditions, to some extent, check their flow.

The sight of attractive food, as we all know, "makes the mouth water," that is, it calls forth the saliva which contains one of the digestive ferments. Thus, at the beginning of a meal, favorable conditions for digestion are established. The saliva, however, acts only upon starch; and, moreover, its action upon this carbohydrate is weak unless the food is thoroughly chewed and mixed in the mouth. Most of us, perhaps, overlook the importance of mastication, which not only crushes all the food-stuffs, preparing them for efficient digestion, but also stimulates the flow of the digestive juices. Furthermore, by thoroughly masticating our food, we know intuitively when we have had enough, and thus avoid overeating.

In the stomach the digestion of starch is continued for a time, but the chief work of gastric digestion concerns the proteins. They alone are attacked by pepsin, a ferment secreted by the mucous membrane of the stomach. Moreover, since pepsin is able to act only when an acid is present, the gastric mucous membrane also secretes hydrochloric acid.

Just as the digestive glands in the neighborhood of the mouth become more active when we are conscious that desirable food is at hand, so do the glands in the stomach. Mastication also stimulates the flow of the gastric juice, and this flow is greater if we enjoy what we eat. Furthermore, it has been shown that, after entrance into the stomach, the food itself increases the flow of the digestive juices. All articles of food are not, however, equally efficient in producing this effect: thus meat requires more pepsin for satisfactory digestion than bread, and consequently meat calls forth a larger quantity of gastric juice.

Fat in all probability is not digested in the stomach; even starch and protein are not broken down sufficiently by the time gastric digestion is complete to permit them to be absorbed into the body. "The value of digestion in the stomach," as Howell says, "is not so much in its own action as in its combined action with that which takes place in the intestine." It is even possible for satisfactory digestion to take place without the assistance of the stomach. This fact has been substantiated by several cases in which men have lived for years after the stomach was removed to eradicate a disease. It is true, nevertheless, that intestinal digestion can be performed more economically if it begins where gastric digestion normally leaves off.

Of the changes wrought in the food by the various digestive processes, those which are the most profound take place in the intestine. While the food is being moved through this organ--some thirty feet in length--it is reduced to simple chemical fragments, which are absorbed by the intestinal wall. Digestion in the intestine is carried on through the agency of a number of ferments, the more important of which are supplied in the juice manufactured by the pancreas. The pancreatic secretion contains three separate and distinct ferments, which act respectively upon carbohydrate, protein, and fat. The absorption of fat, however, is materially assisted also by the action of the bile.

A part of what we eat always escapes digestion; the unused portion, it has been estimated, is somewhat less than one-tenth of an ordinary mixed diet. The residue from vegetables is notably larger than the residue from meat. The undigested portions of all the food- stuffs collect in the lowermost portion of the intestine and form a part of the feces. Here also are gathered the indigestible material we have eaten, the products of bacterial decomposition in the intestine, and other waste substances that the body should throw off.

HOW MUCH FOOD IS NEEDED DURING PREGNANCY?--In connection with the development of the child we have already referred to the difference in the purpose of the constructive processes which go on in the earlier months of gestation and those which take place in the later months. In a general way the first half of pregnancy is occupied with the formation of the embryo from relatively simple structural elements, the second half with its growth into an infant, which acquires ninety per cent. of its substance and weight at birth after the fifth month of embryonic development. A similar contrast may be observed in the nutritional processes of the mother. Often, at the beginning of pregnancy, the appetite is poor and there is indisposition of one kind or another, with the natural result that there is slight if any change in the mother's weight; whereas later a period ensues when her appetite increases, her health improves, and she gains in weight.

Since it is natural that the weight of the mother should remain practically stationary during the early months of pregnancy, it is clear that a diet which has previously been ample will likewise be sufficient for some time after conception has taken place. To most persons, however, it is not clear that the quantity of food ordinarily eaten will suffice also during the later months of pregnancy. On the contrary, popular opinion holds that the prospective mother "should eat for two." It is not unimportant to point out the erroneous character of this superstition, because overeating during pregnancy is much more likely to provoke discomfort than insufficient nourishment.

In order to comprehend the nutritional needs of the prospective mother, one must keep in mind the fact that our food always serves two purposes. These are, as we have seen, to build or to repair tissue and to furnish heat and energy. Since these needs of the body during pregnancy--as at all other times--are best understood when considered in their relation to the food-stuffs which supply them, we shall take up these various ingredients separately.

Protein, which repairs tissue and also furnishes the substance from which new tissue is made, is used more economically during pregnancy than when the maternal functions are inactive. As a result of this economy the same allowance of protein which is sufficient before conception is sufficient also during pregnancy. This fact has been put in the clearest light by extensive observations made upon animals. Dogs which were not pregnant, for example, have been carefully fed so that their food should contain just enough protein to cover the needs of the body and keep their weight constant. Subsequently, when these animals became pregnant precisely the same amount of protein was fed to them. The result was that they gained in weight, and at the same time the waste products of protein they threw off were notably diminished. Such observations, of which there have been a large number yielding concordant results, may be safely taken to mean that an amount of protein previously satisfactory for the animal is also sufficient for her during pregnancy. We are forced to conclude that protein was used more sparingly in the latter condition--a view which has been repeatedly confirmed with regard to human beings as well as animals. It is found, for example, that an amount of protein competent to meet the needs of a man of a given weight will not only provide for the wants of a woman of equal weight while she is pregnant, but will also leave a surplus sufficient for the growth of the fetus.

With regard to the mineral substances, likewise investigations indicate that the "housekeeping" of the body during pregnancy proceeds along unusually economic lines. It is not advisable, therefore, to make any change in the diet with regard to these substances. Attempts have been made to cut down the amount of minerals in the food for the purpose of softening the fetal skeleton. The success sometimes attributed to these efforts is, however, very doubtful, for we know that the mother's tissues will be robbed of minerals for the embryo whenever her food fails to contain them in sufficient amount for her own needs and those of the child. Practically speaking, the mineral content of diet during pregnancy requires no thought, for so long as meat and vegetables are eaten in satisfactory quantity the mineral nutrition will take care of itself.

The food-stuffs which supply heat and energy, since the amount of energy utilized by the body during the latter months of pregnancy is somewhat in excess of that previously required, do not follow the same rule as the protein and the mineral matter. It has been found that just before the fetus becomes mature the energy requirements of the mother are approximately one-fifth greater than in the non- pregnant condition. It is certain, however, that no extra demand for energy exists until the fifth or sixth month of pregnancy, and that the excessive requirement is extremely small until the last three or four weeks. Even then the prospective mother requires less energy- giving food than the average man.

Since the body handles carbohydrate more readily than fat, it is preferable that whatever additional energy pregnancy necessitates should be supplied by carbohydrates. An increase in the daily consumption of fatty food, over and above that previously found agreeable, is not only unnecessary but undesirable. Every-day experience teaches that less fat taken with the meals promotes the comfort of the prospective mother. A glass of rich milk a little before meal time, however, not only makes up for this omission but also prevents "heart-burn," a very common ailment of pregnancy.

Although there is an appreciable increase in the quantity of starch and sugar utilized toward the end of pregnancy, it is generally quite unnecessary to increase these materials correspondingly in the diet. Nearly everyone eats more of all the food-stuffs than the body needs. In the case of the prospective mother the surplus ordinarily taken meets every need incident to her additional energy requirements. Because we eat more than we need, someone has said, with as much truth as humor, that prospective mothers "neither want nor need to eat for two. The fact is more likely that enough for one is too much for two." For the average woman it is wiser to take less during pregnancy rather than more, for over-indulgence is apt to lead to indigestion. The moment when the appetite is satisfied should be accepted as the stopping point, and that will be instinctively recognized if one eats deliberately, and thoroughly masticates the food.

Regularity in the hour of eating is always healthful, and for some prospective mothers three meals a day prove quite satisfactory. Not a few, however, who adhere to this habit make the mistake of eating more than is wise; and large meals are particularly inappropriate to pregnancy. On this account most prospective mothers will be more comfortable if they take some simple and wholesome nourishment at fixed times between meals. Such an arrangement modifies a ravenous appetite, and it is, at the same time, beneficial to those who are not inclined to eat enough at the regular meals. If small amounts of food are taken five or six times a day, a tendency to be nauseated, which is not uncommon in the early months of pregnancy, can often be averted. In the latter months, too, because the capacity of the stomach is diminished through the encroachment of the enlarged womb, frequent meals generally contribute toward comfort and health. While the inevitable consequences of overloading the stomach are to be avoided at all times of the day, it is especially important to remember the disagreeable results of a hearty meal at night. The evening meal should be a light one and should be eaten three or four hours before going to bed.

THE IMPORTANCE OF LIQUID NOURISHMENT.--Every prospective mother should have brought to her attention the great importance of drinking water at regular times and in larger quantities than was formerly her custom. Since water constitutes two-thirds of the substance of our bodies, it is necessary, of course, for everyone; but during pregnancy it is especially necessary for the building of new tissue and for safeguarding the mother's kidneys. Prospective mothers would protect themselves against a number of ailments if they were more careful to drink a sufficient amount of liquids. They may easily determine whether they are doing so, for whenever the urine passed during twenty-four hours measures less than a quart, they are not drinking enough. Generally the daily elimination of urine fluctuates between two and three pints; a larger amount, however, is rather a favorable indication than the reverse.

The variations in the quantity of liquids that healthy persons drink make it impossible to say just how much anyone should take. It may be said with confidence, however, that women who are pregnant should consume at least three quarts of fluid every day, and by far the greater portion of this should be water. The rest may be taken in the form of milk, soup, cocoa, and chocolate. Against the moderate use of tea and coffee no valid objection can be raised; the tradition that they may cause miscarriage is incorrect. For well-known reasons the habitual use of strong tea or coffee is always harmful, and it is, therefore, equally as objectionable during pregnancy as at other times. Beverages which contain a small percentage of alcohol, such as malt and beer, may or may not be helpful; they should be regarded as medicine, not to be taken without consulting a physician.

THE CHOICE OF FOOD.--There is no diet specifically adapted to the state of pregnancy; the prospective mother may usually exercise the same freedom as anyone else in the selection of food. She should, however, choose what will agree with her and avoid that which she cannot digest and assimilate. Personal experience in the main must guide everyone as to what to eat, and most women may follow the dictates of appetite after they become pregnant as safely as they did before.

It is true, of course, that careful scientific observations have taught not only what the nutritional requirements of the body are, but also how the diet may be arranged to satisfy these requirements most conscientiously and economically. "Caloric Feeding" is the name given the method which aims to furnish an individual the exact amount of food, and usually to furnish it at a minimum cost. Its principles are of great practical importance to the commissary of an army or to the purveyor of an institution which provides for large numbers of people; but it is neither necessary nor advisable that the diet of any healthy individual be regulated solely with a view to satisfying the actual requirements of his or her body. Food should possess other qualities than fuel value: first of all it must be appetizing, for appetizing food receives the most thorough digestion.

We all know how variable are our appetites. What appeals to one will not appeal to another, and frequently the same person has no appetite to-day for food that she will eat with relish to-morrow. Precise rules, therefore, to guide healthy persons in the selection of their food are not obtainable; neither are they desirable, for the exercise of individual preference possesses notable advantages. In order, however, that there may not also be disadvantages, the prospective mother, like anyone else, must be content to choose food that is simple, wholesome, and of such a character that it will not throw an undue burden upon the digestive organs.

During pregnancy some uncooked food should be eaten every day. Ripe fruit answers the purpose admirably. At all seasons of the year fruit of one variety or another, such as apples, peaches, apricots, pears, oranges, figs, cherries, pineapples, grapes, plums, strawberries, raspberries, and blackberries may be obtained and should have a place in the diet. In making a choice personal taste alone need be consulted.

Fruit contains a large proportion of water as compared with other articles of diet; and, therefore, is especially capable of quenching thirst. Fruit also lessens the desire for sweets, acts as a laxative, and furnishes mineral material which the body needs. Its laxative effect is most pronounced when it is eaten alone, as, for example, in the morning before breakfast or at night upon going to bed; cooked fruit taken with the meals acts much less effectively. Fruit and vegetable salads are wholesome, but cannot be recommended indiscriminately during pregnancy, for not infrequently the dressing used with them causes discomfort. Under these circumstances it is obvious that one should do without salads.

The cereals wheat, corn, rye, oats, and barley are the most prominent source of starch in an ordinary diet. Breakfast foods manufactured from grain are not only nutritious in themselves, but their value is increased by the milk or cream used with them. Bread is the staple starch-containing food in this country, and starch is our main source of energy, but it is necessary to eat only a small quantity of bread, if the diet includes a relatively large amount of vegetables. It is advantageous to use bread made from unbolted flour (Graham bread) or from corn meal, because the coarse undigested residue which they leave stimulates the movements of the intestine and assists in overcoming the constipation which is generally associated with pregnancy. Pastry must be avoided by those who suffer from indigestion; and every prospective mother should eat pastry only occasionally, and not very much of it at any time. The best desserts are raw and freshly cooked fruit, preserves, gelatin, custard, ice cream, and light puddings, such as rice and tapioca.

Vegetables should be abundant in the diet of every prospective mother. Some of them, however, are digested with difficulty, and on this account cabbage, cauliflower, corn, egg-plant, cucumbers, and radishes should be eaten sparingly. Occasionally it will be necessary to exclude them from the diet altogether. Other vegetables produce flatulence, and for that reason parsnips and beans may cause discomfort. The prejudice, however, which exists against onions, asparagus, and celery should not be heeded; all of them are harmless, and celery thoroughly cooked with milk is very wholesome. Besides these, moreover, there are many highly nutritious and easily digestible vegetables which can be freely recommended, such as both sweet and white potatoes, rice, peas, lima beans, tomatoes, beets, carrots, string beans, spinach, Brussels sprouts, and lettuce.

Vegetable food contains all the material necessary to sustain life, and some persons prefer to adhere strictly to a vegetarian diet. Most prospective mothers, however, find a mixed diet more agreeable, and this is sufficient reason for using it. Furthermore, no fair objection can be raised against the use of animal food, provided the pregnancy is normal. It is important, nevertheless, to remember that meat contains protein in concentrated amounts, and that meat once a day answers every need not only of the mother but also of the growing fetus.

The ideal animal foods are milk and eggs; they contain every ingredient necessary to repair old and to form new tissues. But usually the prospective mother may have any animal food she wishes: beef, veal, lamb, poultry, game, fish, oysters, and clams. The relatively large fat-content of pork, goose, and duck renders them indigestible for some persons, who, of course, should not eat them.

From what we have learned about foods in general and their relation to pregnancy it is clear that the question so often asked by prospective mothers, "Are there any special directions regarding my diet?" may be briefly answered as follows: Under no circumstances is the need of food increased in the first half of pregnancy. During the last two or three months, while the most notable growth of the fetus is in progress, there is a perceptible increase in the amount of energy expended by the mother, and this may be readily supplied by a glass of milk or some equally simple nourishment between meals. Furthermore, throughout pregnancy, most women are made most comfortable by frequent small meals; they will almost certainly suffer discomfort if heavy meals are eaten three times a day.

The most nearly ideal diet consists of very little meat and a comparatively rich allowance of vegetables and fruit. The food should be chosen with regard to individual appetite and should be varied frequently. Thorough mastication always increases the efficiency of a diet. Thus the food will be most perfectly mixed with saliva and broken into fragments which can be readily attacked by the digestive juices of the stomach and the intestines.

CRAVINGS.--There is a well-known tradition that women who are pregnant are subject to longings for one article of diet or another, and that unless the desire be promptly gratified the child will be "marked." In the light of what has already been said regarding maternal impressions, this evidently is nonsense. A prospective mother, like anyone else, does frequently desire one article of food more than another. So long as the object of her wish is not obviously harmful, it should be granted; but if it is not granted no harm will come to the child.

Remarkable instances in which disgusting substances have been craved and eaten are often talked about and have even found their way into popular novels. The unfortunate victims of these unnatural cravings are not of sound mind. With reference to them a physician of unusually broad experience wrote fifty years ago, "I have never met with any example of this sort; which leads me to infer that these longings are more frequent in books than in the practice of our art." This conclusion is even more fully justified to-day than when originally expressed.

THE RELATION BETWEEN THE MOTHER'S DIET AND THE SIZE OF THE CHILD.--
With the beginning of careful, scientific study of the nutritional problems of
pregnancy, investigators were interested to learn the source of the material
which was used to build up the child's body. Two possibilities suggested
themselves: one that the material came from the mother's food and the
other that it was derived from her own flesh. In order to determine which of
these methods was the natural one, animal experimentation was resorted to
and gave identical results in the hands of independent observers. It was
found, as I have already stated, that the same diet which had previously kept
an animal's weight constant was sufficient to meet her requirements during
pregnancy and also to provide for the growth of her offspring. The mother
animal was actually found somewhat heavier at the termination of pregnancy
than at the beginning. It seemed fair to conclude, therefore, that nutrition
had proceeded along more economic lines, and that under these conditions
the customary diet had furnished the material for the formation of the young.
Still other observations indicated that, if the food is not sufficient for both
mother and offspring, it is Nature's plan to protect the young and leave the
mother's wants incompletely satisfied. On the other hand, when an
unnecessarily large amount of nourishment is taken, the excess is stored
partly in the young, and partly in the mother's body.

There can be no doubt that the results of such observations upon animals
are applicable to human beings. Everyone familiar with the practice of
obstetrics knows that women who gratify enormous appetites during
pregnancy, especially if they also fail to take exercise, give birth to large
children. On the other hand, it is said that children born during times of
famine are frequently delivered prematurely, or, if mature, they are small and
puny. A similar though much less marked contrast exists between the babies
of the working classes and the well-to-do, and clearly indicates that the
weight of the baby varies directly with the food of the mother.

The quantity of the food is more influential than its quality, though the latter
is also a factor in determining the size of the child. An excessive amount of
starch or sugar in the mother's diet is stored as fat in the child. On this
account it is reasonable to eat sparingly of candy, cake, and other sweets; but
further attempts to reduce the weight of the fetus by discrimination against

different articles of food are not advisable.

The various theories that have been advanced with a view to reducing the size of the child are impracticable; some of them, rigidly carried out, would actually jeopardize the health of both beings. All of them are designed to make the infant's bones soft and to diminish the fat in its body. To this end, generally about two months before the expected date of birth, the mother's diet is arranged to consist chiefly of meat; and as far as possible she is denied candy, sweet desserts, soup, bread, cereals, vegetables, and water. Such a diet overlooks, among other things, the tremendous importance of liquids to the woman who is pregnant. Certainly its indiscriminate use would result in far more harm than good; and no one should adopt it without minute directions from a physician.

Attempts to make the infant's bones soft by limiting the mother to food containing extremely small amounts of lime and other minerals are also unnatural, for we have learned that whenever the mother's food fails to contain the material the fetus requires the mother's tissues are called upon to supply it. Under these conditions, therefore, her bones will give up their lime.

It is of the very first importance that the mother's nourishment be correct from the standpoint of her own requirements, and such treatment will also redound most beneficially to the child. She should never fall, however, into the error of over-eating, which will not benefit her and will cause unnecessary growth of the fetus. On the other hand, there can be no justification for measures that tend to weaken her. She may be careful, in other words, to avoid over- growth of the fetus, but should not adopt a diet so restricted as to interfere with normal development. So long as her health is successfully maintained, she may give herself no concern as to what the size of the child is likely to be. That is a detail which concerns her physician, and which will be observed by him several weeks before the expected date of birth.

CHAPTER V

THE CARE OF THE BODY

The Bowels--The Kidneys--The Skin--Bathing--Douches--Clothing-- Corsets--The Breasts.

If we stop to think it is only too apparent that the human body is a machine. We seize energy in one form and convert it into another, just as truly as do the windmill, the locomotive, and the dynamo. In the case of the human machine, the latent energy of the food is turned into the various activities of everyday life. Our bodies utilize their fuel more perfectly than any machine that man has invented; but they fail, nevertheless, to do so completely. And just as the efficiency of an engine cannot be maintained unless the smoke escapes and the ashes are raked away, so no human being can enjoy health unless his waste products are promptly removed. The task of removal, as most of us know, is assumed by our excretory organs, which include the bowels, the kidneys, the skin, and the lungs.

During pregnancy the mother must get rid not only of her own waste products, but also of those of the child. The waste products of the child, if weighed, would not amount to a great deal; but they are by no means negligible. So far as we can tell, it is chiefly on account of their peculiar character that they increase the work of the mother's excretory organs. Whatever the cause, they do increase it, and experience has taught us that these organs must always be kept in a healthful condition to protect both the mother and the child from harm. Consequently a prospective mother who wishes to take proper care of her body must, in the first place, direct her attention toward keeping up the normal activity of all the excretory functions.

THE BOWELS.--While pregnant, nine out of ten women suffer from mild constipation. Those who have been previously troubled with this complaint may find it aggravated from the outset, but in most instances it does not appear until after several months have passed. Constipation is explained by the fact that the enlarged womb presses against the intestines; and, as the enlargement increases, constipation generally becomes more pronounced. No doubt there was a time when women, perhaps unconsciously, counteracted this natural result of pregnancy by the use of a diet consisting largely of fruit and vegetables and also by outdoor exercise. Such measures, indeed, still afford the simplest means of overcoming constipation.

Throughout pregnancy the bowels should move at least once every day.

When they do not, some of the waste material that should be removed is absorbed by the body and seeks to leave it through the organs that are already doing their full share of work. For example, under such conditions, the kidneys, instead of exerting themselves more vigorously, may become less active than they were.

It is everyone's duty to form the habit of having the bowels move regularly. Now the most favorable opportunity for assisting the intestines to empty themselves occurs shortly after meal-time, since the involuntary movements of the intestines are most active while digestion is in progress. It should be regarded as an imperative duty, therefore, to grant Nature such an opportunity every morning just after breakfast. This should be done at a definite hour, day after day, even though the inclination is absent; and in many instances the desired habit will be formed.

A glass of water on going to bed or on getting up has a laxative effect; and there are other dietary measures which may be employed with advantage. Thus, coarseness of the food, as we know, stimulates intestinal activity, and this fact explains the peculiar value of Graham bread, bran bread, and corn bread. Fresh fruit and vegetables counteract constipation for two reasons, namely, because they leave in the bowels a relatively large amount of undigested substance, and because they contain ingredients that have a specific purgative action. Such ingredients are especially noteworthy in rhubarb, tomatoes, apples, peaches, pears, figs, prunes, and berries.

Enemas used as a routine measure are mischievous. They interfere with the "tone" of the bowel-muscle so that it acts sluggishly and bring about a condition in which the bowels will not move without artificial stimulation. At best these irrigations remove no more than the contents of the lower bowel, and should be employed only when there is acute and urgent need of clearing out the rectum.

Obstinate constipation is uncommon, and strong purgatives are seldom needed. If they become necessary, a physician should be consulted as to what to take. Whenever dietary measures and exercise, which is discussed in the next chapter, fail to counteract the natural tendency toward constipation, the prospective mother may generally resort to "senna prunes" or some equally simple and harmless household remedy. Senna prunes are prepared as follows: Place an ounce of dried senna leaves in a jar and pour a quart of boiling water on them. Allow to stand two or three hours; strain off the leaves and throw them away. To the liquor add a pound of prunes. Cover and place on the back of the stove, allowing to simmer until half the liquor has boiled away. Add a pint of water and sweeten to taste, preferably with brown sugar. The prunes should be eaten with the evening meal. The number required must be learned from experience. Begin with half a dozen, and increase or decrease the number, as required. The syrup is an even stronger laxative than the prunes.

THE KIDNEYS.--Any one may judge for herself whether or not the bowels are doing their work satisfactorily, but not so with the kidneys. For this purpose the urine must be examined by a physician. In spite of this fact, considerable responsibility rests upon the prospective mother, whose duty it is to collect the specimens properly--a detail that is apt to be neglected. It is impossible to urge too strongly the importance of saving, at regular intervals, all the urine passed in twenty-four hours, of protecting it from decomposition, and of sending a sample to the physician. The intervals may be longer at first, for the kidneys have very little extra work to do until the sixth month. Usually, therefore, it is a satisfactory plan to send a sample for analysis the first of each month during the early half of pregnancy; but during the latter half one should be sent the first and the fifteenth of each month.

To estimate the exact amount of urine passed in twenty-four hours and to protect it properly, in the first place, the vessel in which it will be collected should be carefully scalded out. As a further precaution against decomposition, add a teaspoonful of chloroform to the vessel, which should be kept covered, and not allowed to stand in a warm room. Unless these details are conscientiously observed, putrefaction may take place and vitiate the analysis the physician wishes to make. The precise amount of urine which the kidneys excrete in twenty-four hours will be determined as follows: At a convenient time, for example at 8 A.M., empty the bladder and throw the urine away; this marks the beginning of the observation. Subsequently, save all the urine passed during the day and night, and finally at 8 o'clock the next morning empty the bladder and add this urine to that previously collected. The total amount, thus collected, should be measured.

It is unnecessary to send all the urine to the physician; six ounces, somewhat less than half a pint, will be enough. But the physician should know what the total amount was found to be; therefore, a record of the measurement, the date, and the patient's name should accompany the sample. If limited to a single fact about the urine, it would be most helpful to know the amount passed during the twenty- four hours. In this way, as I have already pointed out, the patient herself may derive valuable information, for if the urine is scanty in amount--that is, less than a quart--she should drink more water.

Unscrupulous newspaper advertisements alarm people through incorrect statements about trouble with the kidneys. For example, they declare that a sediment in the urine is a sign of disease; but that is false. The mere act of cooling sometimes causes substances to crystallize out of perfectly normal urine. Or, putrefactive changes which frequently take place after the urine has stood for a time may cause some of its normal constituents to be precipitated. A sediment, either white, pink, or yellow, may indicate that the urine is too concentrated, and consequently means that the individual should drink water more freely; but it generally means nothing more serious. The really important abnormal constituents of the urine, namely, albumin and sugar, never form a sediment.

"Pain in the back" is a complaint frequently used to defraud the public. This symptom does not indicate Bright's disease. It is generally due to the muscles far away from the kidneys, with which, usually, the pain has nothing whatever to do. Similarly a desire to pass the urine frequently does not indicate any disturbance of kidney function, but is explained by the pressure of the enlarged womb against the bladder; it is a very annoying, yet a natural, result of pregnancy.

THE SKIN.--The functions of the skin are at the very foundation of health. It protects the delicate structures which it covers, assists in the regulation of the temperature of the body, and excretes waste products. The excretory function of the skin is always active, but we are unconscious of this activity except on warm days and at times when we perspire freely. In the coldest weather, however, the body throws off what physiologists call the "insensible perspiration." The most important measures for the care of the skin are those intended to insure the activity of the sweat glands, namely, bathing and proper clothing. But before considering these measures, we will describe certain alterations in the skin which cannot escape the notice of the prospective mother, and which she is likely to misinterpret.

On account of the growth of the uterus the abdominal wall is stretched during pregnancy. To a certain degree the skin yields to the distention, but it finally cracks, and lines appear which are commonly called "pregnancy streaks." At first they are delicate and pink or blue in color; later they become white and more extensive.

The streaks indicate the situation of small breaks in the deeper layer of the skin, which is less elastic than the upper layer. They are not painful, and should never cause anxiety. Their size and number vary with the degree of abdominal distention, which in turn depends upon various factors, such as the size of the child and the quantity of amniotic fluid. Although these streaks are most frequently located upon the lower part of the abdomen, they may extend to the outer sides of the thighs; and occasionally appear over the breasts, since they too enlarge during pregnancy. Stretching of the skin, of course, is not confined to pregnancy; consequently, the same kind of streaks often appear in people who are growing stout.

Attempts to prevent or limit the pregnancy streaks prove futile. There is a common belief that they may be prevented by the use of vaselin, goose-grease, mutton-fat, or some one of a variety of lotions; but this teaching is not borne out by experience. None of these applications, however, are harmful, and there can be no objection to using them except that they cause needless soiling of the clothing. After the child is born the streaks fade of their own accord, though they rarely disappear entirely.

In certain localities the skin grows darker during pregnancy. We have already referred to the deepening of the color around the nipple as one of the signs of pregnancy; a similar but much less pronounced discoloration occurs about the navel, which also becomes shallow and may begin to pout in the latter months of pregnancy. About this time, with very few exceptions, there appears a more or less intense brown line which runs downward from the navel in the middle of the abdomen. Sometimes, though not very often, small dark areas, which have been called "liver spots," appear elsewhere over the body. The name is unfortunate, for the spots do not indicate a disorder of the liver.

At present it is generally admitted that alterations in the color of the skin during pregnancy are due to deposits of iron. This mineral substance, among others, as we have learned, is required for the development of the embryo. The child is born with a supply of iron calculated to meet its needs for about a year. Such a reserve is necessary, as Bunge has pointed out, because human milk does not contain enough iron to satisfy the infant's requirements. During pregnancy, therefore, the mother's blood transports iron to the placenta, where it can be absorbed into the child's system; and while being thus transported some of it is deposited in the maternal tissues. The deposits are especially frequent, as I have mentioned, in the middle line of the abdomen, on account of the arrangement of the blood vessels there. Deposits elsewhere may depend upon other conditions; but whatever their cause the pigmentation vanishes a short time after the birth.

Alterations in the color of the skin have no effect upon its excretory function, which, indeed, generally becomes more active during pregnancy. According to one estimate, the average person possesses twenty-eight miles of sweat glands. If these figures are not sufficient to demonstrate the importance of the skin as an excretory organ, surely no one will fail to be impressed by the tragic result which in one case followed throwing all the sweat glands out of action. This was brought about in the case of a young boy whose body was covered with gold leaf to provide entertainment at a Parisian festival. The living statue was not exhibited, however, for shortly after the youth was gilded he became ill and died.

In health more than a pint of water is eliminated through the skin every day, and along with it waste products are removed from the body. Exercise, hot drinks, warm weather, and heavy clothing promote the activity of the sweat glands. Under certain circumstances physicians endeavor to relieve the kidneys by stimulating their patients to perspire freely. It should be clear, therefore, that when a prospective mother naturally perspires it is a good indication. Attempts to stop the perspiration are always ill advised; rather should this function be encouraged by keeping the skin in good condition with baths and warm clothing.

BATHING.--The accumulation of dead skin, grease, dust, and dried perspiration on the surface of the body hinders the actions of the sweat glands. Some of this material is wiped off by the clothing, and more of it is removed by washing with plain water; but the most effectual cleansing results from a liberal use of warm water and soap.

Since the prospective mother must throw off the waste products of the embryo as well as those of her own body, it is obvious that cleanliness is never more important than during pregnancy. For this reason she should take a tepid tub bath or shower every day. It is not necessary that the temperature of the bath be determined with accuracy or that it be always the same; but generally a temperature between 80 and 90 degrees F. is found most agreeable. At this temperature a bath is termed "indifferent," because it is neither stimulating nor depressing; it is employed purely for cleansing the body. Every part of the body should be well soaped, and from ten to fifteen minutes should be given to washing all the exposed surfaces. The best time for such a bath is just before going to bed, though there is no objection to taking it during the day, provided that two hours have passed since the last meal, and that another hour is permitted to elapse before one goes out of doors or undertakes anything that requires exertion.

Prolonged hot baths are fatiguing. They draw the blood from the interior to the surface of the body; and during pregnancy they are particularly depressing. Vapor and steam baths have a similar action and should never be taken without the consent of a physician. They serve admirably for the treatment of rare complications of pregnancy; but, like medicine, their use should be limited to cases in which they are clearly indicated.

Unless disagreeable results are noticed, those who have become accustomed to cold baths may continue to take them during pregnancy, but others should not. If, however, the temperature of the water is modified so that it will not produce a shock, no one need omit the morning plunge or shower which most persons find invigorating. Sponging answers the same purpose, for the intent of the morning bath is not to cleanse the body but to arouse the circulation. A thorough rub-down assists in bringing the blood to the surface of the body. Bath and massage together thus constitute a kind of skin gymnastics especially beneficial throughout pregnancy.

Although hot foot-baths have sometimes been thought to cause miscarriage, there is no good reason for believing they ever do. Sea- bathing, on the contrary, may be directly responsible for such a mishap. It is true that pregnant women sometimes indulge in surf- bathing without harmful results; nevertheless the danger of miscarriage they assume is not slight. The shock of the low temperature, the exertion required to keep a firm footing, and the pounding of the surf against the abdomen are all unfavorable influences which more than counterbalance any advantage of such a bath. On the other hand, there is slight risk if any in bathing in a quiet stream or lake.

DOUCHES.--A great many women have the conviction that the vagina is not clean and should, therefore, be regularly cleansed by means of irrigations. This assumption is false and the treatment based upon it is unnecessary. In structure the walls of the vagina closely resemble the skin, but unlike the skin they do not contain glands; the vagina, therefore, has nothing to do with the elimination of waste products from the body. The secretion which issues from the vagina really originates in the glands around the mouth of the womb, and serves to protect the birth-canal against infection from harmful bacteria.

Careful examinations have shown that under normal conditions, which of course include pregnancy, disease-producing bacteria are absent from the vagina; in this respect the vagina is even cleaner than the skin, for disease-producing bacteria are present on the surface of the body. The vaginal secretion becomes more abundant during pregnancy, and the increase is interpreted as an additional guarantee against infection at the time of labor. So far as possible, therefore, this natural antiseptic should not be disturbed.

The advice to abstain from douches will not be adopted by every prospective mother without protest, for, as I have said, many women regard them as necessary to cleanliness. Others who have delicate skins are occasionally annoyed by the irritation of the vaginal secretion, which is not only increased during pregnancy but has a more pronouncedly acid character. Under extraordinary circumstances, it may be permissible to use douches in the early part of pregnancy, but it is practically never advisable to do so during the month preceding the expected date of confinement. Furthermore, at no time should the use of douches be begun without consulting a physician.

A more rational hygienic measure for the relief of itching and smarting about the vaginal orifice consists in removing the secretion as soon as it appears. In other words, the external parts should be kept clean and dry. Great comfort is often derived from the use of a "sitz-bath," which may be easily prepared by placing a small tub upon a low stool and pouring in warm water (about 90 degrees F.) until it is five or six inches deep. Cold sitz-baths are useful in the treatment of hemorrhoids. Whether the bath be hot or cold, the treatment should continue from ten to fifteen minutes, and after it the skin should be thoroughly dried.

A special form of tub, called a "bidet," has been devised to facilitate bathing the parts in question. The device is convenient but expensive, and is certainly not essential. Every purpose will be served by the small tub, provided the desired temperature of the bath is properly maintained by changing the water as may be necessary.

CLOTHING.--In these days at least it is not idle to remark that the first use of clothes is to keep the body warm; all other services they are made to perform are secondary and relatively unimportant. There are very good reasons, to be sure, for dressing neatly and even for dressing in accord with the fashion, so long as the prevailing styles are not harmful. Odd as it may seem, these are matters which are not without significance for the physical well-being of a prospective mother. Neat and comfortable clothing will help her to overcome a natural inclination to become a "stay-at-home," and on this account an inconspicuous way of dressing is often more valuable than medicine. So long as they do not attract attention, most prospective mothers go out in the day time, mingle with their acquaintances, and attend public places of amusement. Deference to fashion, therefore, may contribute substantially to good health.

Yet no prospective mother can afford to forget that first of all her clothing must keep the body warm. Our clothing confines a cushion of air which prevents the escape of the heat that we generate. Now, since dry air conducts heat poorly and moist air conducts it readily, the underclothes should be made of material that absorbs the perspiration; otherwise the heat that the body generates is quickly lost. Woolen garments effectually absorb the perspiration and should be given the preference. Most persons who cannot wear wool next the skin must choose cotton, since silk and linen are much more expensive; there is not in this, however, a serious deprivation. Cotton undergarments are perfectly hygienic; adapting their weight to the season of the year, one will find them equally satisfactory in summer and winter.

Except in summer every inch of the body should be covered with the underclothing; this means that high-neck and long-sleeve shirts and long drawers should be worn, for healthful activity of the skin can thus be best preserved. It is well known to physicians who practice obstetrics that the kidneys fail in their work more frequently during the winter than the summer. To my mind, this is chiefly explained by the way women dress. Even with light clothing the sweat glands respond actively to the heat of summer and thus relieve the kidneys, but in cold weather the sweat glands will not remove their share of the waste products unless the clothing is warm.

Nature generally indicates that the body should be kept warm during pregnancy. Many prospective mothers complain of perspiring freely; others, if reproached because they are not clad warmly enough, reply that they must wear light clothing to keep from perspiring. Thus they discount or render absolutely ineffective a most important natural safeguard against serious complications. It cannot be too strongly emphasized that warm clothing helps to maintain healthful activity of the kidneys quite as much as a proper amount of exercise and the drinking of a suitable quantity of water.

The texture of the outer garments should take into account this same quality of warmth; in other respects in selecting them personal taste is an excellent guide. Outfitters carry a variety of maternity garments; patterns for such garments are also sold by dealers, so that those who cannot afford the ready-made clothes will find it easy to have them made at home. Alterations in the clothing are compulsory as pregnancy advances, and should be timely, made in anticipation of inevitable development rather than in response to it. No prospective mother need go to the extreme of "Reform Clothes"; her apparel should illustrate both her good sense and her personal pride.

It is obviously even more harmful during pregnancy than at other times to cramp the body by the clothing; the chest and the abdomen, the parts most likely to be compressed, are at such times most in need of freedom. To a slight degree natural causes always compress the chest from below upward; and on this account nothing should be allowed to hamper the expansion of the lungs from side to side. On the other hand, if the waist is constricted, not the breathing movements alone but also the growth of the womb will be interfered with. In order to avoid such disagreeable consequences, and at the same time to limit the extent of the maternity wardrobe, skirts may be fitted with practical devices which permit letting out the waistband as occasion demands. So far as possible, however, all the clothing should be hung from the shoulders, and under no circumstances should heavy skirts be worn.

Shoes contribute toward health, or the lack of it, more significantly than the average person realizes. It is particularly advisable that prospective mothers should select foot-wear with care, because their bodies are heavier than usual. The feet are apt to become swollen in the latter months of pregnancy, and consequently the shoes should be roomy, but should always fit. To escape the discomfort of tight shoes, it is generally advisable to wear a shoe an inch longer and broader than the foot at rest.

High heels have been proved a frequent cause of back-ache; half of such cases, in all probability, may be thus explained. High heels tilt the body forward in such a way that the erect posture can be maintained only by an unnatural tenseness of the back-muscles. Some strain of this kind is inevitable during the latter months of pregnancy on account of the enlargement and the position of the womb; it is reasonable, therefore, to minimize it by wearing low, broad heels.

Besides being responsible for many cases of backache, high heels add greatly to the danger of tripping and falling; for this reason alone they should not be worn. Improper foot-gear and not the joints themselves deserve the blame for weak ankles. To prevent "turning the ankle," it is not necessary to restrict oneself to high shoes, but merely to see that the shoes that are worn have low heels and broad soles. Such shoes provide a sure, firm footing, and this the prospective mother particularly needs.

CORSETS.--No question connected with women's dress has provoked so much discussion as the use of corsets. "Are corsets necessary to health?" has been differently answered by those who would appear to be equally competent authorities. In the time of our savage ancestors we may safely conclude that they were not used; and, therefore, it is really a question as to whether their continued use for generation after generation has finally made some support of this kind indispensable to the average woman. While that matter has not as yet been settled, it is obvious that custom is really responsible for the conviction of many women that they appear slovenly without corsets. On the other hand, not a few women, unmindful of fashion, never wear them; they testify that they are healthier for doing so. Whether this be true or not, no one can honestly believe that corsets will soon be banished; and the practical problem is to distinguish between those that may do good and those certain to do harm.

During pregnancy the abdomen tends to fall forward and slightly downward, and though it is in pregnancies after the first that this tendency is most marked, every prospective mother will be more comfortable if she wears some sort of support to counteract what physicians term a "pendulous abdomen." Such a condition can be prevented by the use of several appliances, and the device best suited to the case should be chosen. Those who have never become accustomed to corsets will probably find a corset-waist or an abdominal supporter the most comfortable and useful. But the average young woman who has previously employed a sensible, well made, and loosely fitting corset need make no change until the third or fourth month of pregnancy. From then on she should wear a corset especially designed to conform with the changes that naturally occur in the figure.

There is a plan, wrong in principle, which many adopt. Reasoning that it will be necessary to change the corset from time to time, and desiring to practice economy, a number of women purchase the cheapest corset at hand. This they replace with a larger one of the same style from time to time. The result is that an improperly fitting garment is worn continuously; and, in the end, this plan proves almost as expensive as, and far less suitable than, a proper corset, which would remain serviceable throughout pregnancy, or at least until a few weeks before confinement.

Most, and probably all, of the injuries for which corsets are responsible result from their misuse. Naturally serious consequences may be expected if they are worn with the design of compressing the abdomen so as to render pregnancy less noticeable or perhaps to conceal it altogether. Thus worn, the corset becomes not only an instrument of torture but a source of danger both to the mother and to the child. Fortunately there are very few women who fail to appreciate the risk of thus striving to disguise their condition; and generally it is the needless discomfort, the trifling ills thoughtlessly inflicted upon themselves, that prospective mothers must be taught to avoid.

At present there are manufactured a number of excellent maternity corsets; but there are also worthless types, and some likely to do harm. To judge them fairly they must be examined with regard to several requirements. In the first place the corset should not be stiff and should always be capable of easy adjustment; it must never interfere with the activity of any organ. As _enceinte_, the French word meaning pregnant, signifies, the prospective mother should be unbound. Tight clothing, as we have already remarked, hinders the breathing movements; it also interferes with the action of the heart, and occasionally causes the child to assume an unfavorable position within the uterus. The adjustment of the maternity corset to the progressive development of the body is generally provided for by means of extra lacings down the sides, and by the insertion of elastic material.

The maternity corset, in the next place, must support the enlarged uterus. Correctly shaped and worn, it extends well down in front, fits snugly around the hips, and arches forward so as to conform to the curve of the abdomen. In place of the arching, or "cupping" as manufacturers call it, some maternity corsets have attached to their lower edge limp flaps of a strong fabric which lace together. The maternity corset-waist also should extend well under the abdomen and fit snugly around the hips.

Finally, the corset should support the bust; the unpleasant sensations due to congestion of the breasts can be relieved most successfully by elevating them. It is exceedingly important, however, that the upper part of the corset should fit loosely, for otherwise the development of the breasts may be hindered, and the nipples depressed. As a further precaution against pressure above and also to secure the proper amount of support below, it is generally advisable to begin putting on the corset while lying down. In every case the corset should be laced from below upward; if laced in the opposite direction it fails to lift the womb and tends to push all the abdominal organs downward.

Any kind of corset is likely to become uncomfortable toward the end of pregnancy; and of course should then be discarded. An abdominal supporter made of woven linen or rubber is frequently used to advantage during the last three or four weeks. With the first pregnancy the supporter is rarely necessary, but with subsequent ones it is frequently useful as early as the sixth month and is indispensable later. A substitute for the manufactured supporter can be made at home. Some such device often facilitates turning in bed, and on that account may be found even more useful at night than during the day.

THE BREASTS.--Personal hygiene during pregnancy includes the preparation of the breasts with a view to success in nursing. All measures which promote the health of a prospective mother also serve to equip her for the nursing period; and in that sense the directions just given for the care of the body, as well as the rules to follow in the next chapter regarding a wholesome way of living, bear directly upon lactation. But there are also local measures to be adopted, some of which, such as supporting the breasts and avoiding constriction by the clothing, have already been mentioned. Finally, the nipples must be toughened and, if short or flat, they must be drawn out, for the best supply of milk will count for nothing if the infant cannot nurse comfortably.

Some approved method of toughening the nipples so that they will not be injured by the sucking efforts of the infant, no matter how vigorous, should be begun eight weeks before the expected date of confinement; to start earlier will do no harm, but it is quite unnecessary. A number of procedures have been advocated, but in my own experience the following simple method is the best. The nipples are scrubbed for five minutes, night and morning, with soap and warm water. Generally, a soft brush, such as a complexion-brush, is satisfactory; but if this is too harsh, at first a wash cloth may be used. After having been thoroughly scrubbed the nipples are anointed with lanolin and covered with a small square of clean, old linen to prevent soiling of the clothing.

Another method widely used, but somewhat less trustworthy, consists in bathing the nipples and applying a dilute solution of alcohol. Formerly brandy, whiskey, or cologne were recommended, but at present the following solution is commonly used. A tablespoonful of powdered boric acid is added to three ounces of water and thoroughly mixed. This is poured into a six-ounce bottle, which is then filled with grain alcohol (95 per cent). The solution is applied twice a day with a small piece of absorbent cotton.

Well-formed nipples need only be toughened, but depressed nipples require additional treatment; and this should be begun about the middle of pregnancy. The old-fashioned way of making the nipple more prominent was to cover it with the mouth of a bottle which had previously been warmed. The vacuum created, as the bottle cooled, drew the nipple out. Similarly, the bowl of a clay pipe was sometimes placed over the nipple; the patient sucked the stem, the nipple was drawn into the bowl, and with persistence day after day success was often attained. A similar and somewhat more aesthetic procedure is now employed. The nipple is seized between the thumb and finger and alternately pulled out and allowed to retract. These manipulations, if faithfully practiced for several months, generally make the nipple prominent enough for the infant to grasp. Occasionally patients need to wear a contrivance sold at instrument stores which consists of a circular piece of wood modeled to fit the breast and perforated in the middle to accommodate the nipple. The appliance should not be used unless a physician thinks it necessary.

Directions regarding the care of the breasts are sometimes taken lightly, yet such care is not a minor duty. Now and then a patient will pass through pregnancy uneventfully, will be delivered without difficulty, and will enter upon what promises to be a rapid convalescence when her recovery is interrupted by the development of inflammation of the breast. Because such a complication may be prevented, its appearance is the more to be regretted. Furthermore, the responsibility for its prevention usually rests with the patient herself. If she has been conscientious in preparing the nipples and continues to watch them throughout the nursing period, the annoyance of an abscess will almost certainly be prevented.

CHAPTER VI

GENERAL HYGIENIC MEASURES

The Need of Fresh Air--Outdoor Exercise--Massage and Gymnastics--The Influence of Work upon Pregnancy--Relaxation and Rest--Is Traveling Harmful?--Mental Diversion.

Besides the hygienic measures described in the preceding chapter, whose observance should be recognized as more or less obligatory, there are more general questions of conduct, such as exercise, relaxation, mental occupation, and amusement, which are also important. These measures, although frequently determined merely by personal inclination or by the force of circumstances, nevertheless exert a tremendous influence upon health. This fact a prospective mother is likely to realize, for she is certain to consider not only her own welfare but also that of the expected child; and she is consequently concerned about details of conduct that most persons would regard as trivial. She may, indeed, be too conscientious. Well- meaning friends, sometimes in reply to her questions and sometimes without solicitation, offer her a great deal of advice. Their counsel, aside from the fact that some of it may be misleading, may have the effect of prescribing so many rules that, if she followed them all, she would never lose sight of the fact that she is pregnant. Such a degree of self-consciousness is certain to make her unduly apprehensive. The proper attitude of mind is quite the opposite; so far as possible the prospective mother should forget that she is pregnant. This state of mind is really the more rational, for if a woman's daily life has previously been in accord with such simple rules of health as everyone should adopt, the existence of pregnancy calls for very slight changes.

It does not, for example, condemn her to inactivity and seclusion, for it is advisable to lead a moderately active life during pregnancy. Of course, such obvious indiscretions as prolonged exertion, violent exercise, and fatiguing journeys should be avoided, for transgression of the laws of health brings its own punishment, generally in the form of discomfort, more quickly, and often more severely, during pregnancy than at other times. Yet, on the whole, it is more frequently necessary to emphasize to prospective mothers what they should do than what they should avoid. This happens to be the case because, as a rule, they are inclined to become recluses. For fear of attracting attention they often wish to give up outdoor exercise during the day; they stay away from public places of amusement, and deny themselves other pleasures to which they have been accustomed. Against this tendency they must be warned, for if they yield to it they will surely be the worse off both physically and mentally. Every prospective mother should make up her mind to enjoy recreation out of doors regardless of comments.

THE NEED OF PURE AIR.--Outdoor life has been so urgently advocated of late that the public has come to appreciate its benefits almost as fully as do physicians. The existence of pregnancy does not lessen, but rather enhances, the value of fresh air; in order to enjoy the best health during this period one should spend at least two hours out of doors every day. Neither the season of the year nor the state of weather should modify this obligation. If the sun is shining the "airing" is more delightful, but it should be taken in bad weather also, on a protected porch or in a room with the windows wide open.

Even when the injunction to be regularly out of doors is observed women are accustomed to spend the greater portion of the day in the house, and on that account special attention must be given to keeping the air of the house pure. Ventilation takes care of itself in summer, when the windows are open, but in cold weather, when in our anxiety to keep the temperature comfortable we may overlook the need of fresh air, it demands close attention. The necessity of ventilation at all times is due, of course, to the composition of the atmosphere and to the changes produced in it as we breathe.

The air about us is a mixture of gases, of which oxygen and nitrogen are the most important. Although nitrogen, which constitutes four- fifths of the atmosphere, is taken into our lungs in breathing, we make no use of it, but breathe it out in precisely the same condition as we take it in. As chemically combined in the food-stuff known as protein, nitrogen is indispensable to animal life; but our bodies make no use of the gaseous form of nitrogen. Oxygen, on the other hand, supports life; and though it forms less than one-fifth of the atmospheric air, it is present in ample amount for our needs. After we draw air into our lungs, the oxygen it contains is absorbed by the blood and used by the tissues. In return our tissues give up a waste product, carbonic acid gas, which is thrown off by the lungs. It is interesting to observe that the carbonic acid gas which animals exhale supports the life of plants, and that the plants, under the influence of sunlight, give back pure oxygen to the atmosphere. Obviously, the complementary relation exhibited here is of mutual benefit.

The average person uses about four bushels of air a minute. Consequently, rooms that are occupied must be constantly replenished with fresh air; otherwise the point is quickly reached where the occupants are breathing an atmosphere that is not only poor in oxygen but saturated with carbonic acid gas and other impurities conveyed by the breath. Foul air such as this causes headache, dizziness, faintness, nausea, and occasionally even more serious disturbances. Those who live in "close" rooms day after day grow pale and languid; their appetite fails and some of their natural power of resistance against illness is lost. Many people are unhealthy simply because they neglect to supply their living quarters with a steady stream of air from the outside.

While it is impossible to keep the air in any room as pure as the outside atmosphere, perfectly satisfactory ventilation can be easily arranged. Some of the impure air in a house is always escaping of its own accord and its place is taken by air from the outside. Thus, the cracks around the windows and doors let bad air out and good air in; and, besides, most building materials are porous. These natural paths, however, must be supplemented. The simplest device for ventilation, which is also the best, consists in opening a window at the top and bottom. The width of the opening may be regulated so as to permit the air in the room to change without occasioning disagreeable drafts; if necessary the current may be broken by a screen of some pervious material placed in the opening.

The bed-room should always be supplied with plenty, of fresh air, which "quiets the nerves" and helps one to sleep soundly. Furthermore, the temperature of the bed-room should be lower than the temperature of rooms occupied during the day. Both these requisites will be properly met by leaving a window open at night, which may be done throughout the year in most climates, if one puts on enough covering. There is no danger of catching cold from sleeping with the window open; on the contrary, breathing fresh air day and night is one of the best ways to prevent colds.

OUTDOOR EXERCISE.--Outdoor exercise is indispensable to good health. It benefits not only the muscles, but the whole body. By this means the action of the heart is strengthened, and consequently all the tissues receive a rich supply of oxygen. Exercise also promotes the digestion and the assimilation of the food. It stimulates the sweat glands to become more active; and, for that matter, the other excretory organs as well. It invigorates the muscles, strengthens the nerves, and clears the brain. There is, indeed, no part of the human machine that does not run more smoothly if its owner exercises systematically in the open air; and during normal pregnancy there is no exception to this rule. Only in extremely rare cases--those, namely, in which extraordinary precautions must be taken to prevent miscarriage--will physicians prohibit outdoor recreation and, perhaps, every other kind of exertion. Under such circumstances the good effects that most persons secure from exercise should be sought from the use of massage.

The amount of exercise which the prospective mother should take cannot be stated precisely, but what can be definitely said is this-- she should stop the moment she begins to feel tired. Fatigue is only one step short of exhaustion--and, since exhaustion must always be carefully guarded against, the safest rule will be to leave off exercising at a point where one still feels capable of doing more without becoming tired. Women who have laborious household duties to perform do not require as much exercise as those who lead sedentary lives; but they do require just as much fresh air, and should make it a rule to sit quietly out of doors two or three hours every day. It will be found, furthermore, that the limit of endurance is reached more quickly toward the end of pregnancy than at the beginning; a few patients will find it necessary to stop exercise altogether for a week or two before they are delivered.

Walking is the best kind of exercise, but long tramps are inadvisable during pregnancy, except for those who have previously been accustomed to them. Most women who are pregnant find that a two or three-mile walk daily is all they enjoy, and very few are inclined to indulge in six miles, which is generally accepted as the upper limit. Perhaps the best way to measure a walk is by the length of time it consumes. Accordingly, a very sensible plan is to begin with a walk just long enough not to be fatiguing and to increase it by five minutes each day until able to walk an hour without becoming overtired. It is always advisable not to crowd the exercise of a day into a single period but rather to take it in several installments, for example, an hour in the morning, and another in the afternoon. Under all circumstances, it must never be forgotten that the feeling of fatigue is a peremptory signal to stop, no matter how short the walk has been.

Very few outdoor sports can be unconditionally recommended to a prospective mother. Because athletic exercise is either too violent or else jolts or jars the body a great deal, it is especially dangerous in the early months of pregnancy--the only time when it is likely to be at all attractive. Croquet, alone, perhaps, is free from these objections. Although golf and tennis are by no means certain to bring on miscarriage, they involve a risk which, slight though it may perhaps be, will not be assumed by cautious women.

Horseback riding during pregnancy is injurious. We occasionally hear of women who have ridden horseback without immediate harmful consequences, but they have nevertheless exposed themselves to danger unnecessarily. It is better to give up skating and dancing also than to run the risk of accident, especially since these diversions are attended with some danger of falling. In a general way, whenever the question of entering into any kind of recreation must be decided, it is wise to err on the conservative side rather than risk overstepping the limit of endurance and having to pay a penalty more or less severe.

Carriage riding cannot take the place of walking and can scarcely be classed as exercise; it is wholesome, nevertheless, because it takes the participant out of doors and provides a change of scene. Certain details, however, should be carefully observed; thus, a safe horse, a carriage that rides easily, and smooth roads should be selected. Similar advice pertains to motoring; with smooth roads, a cautious driver, and a comfortable machine, short rides in an automobile are not harmful. Carriage riding and motoring are particularly serviceable as a means of getting outdoor diversion during the last few weeks of pregnancy.

MASSAGE AND GYMNASTICS.--If a prospective mother is obliged to stay in bed several weeks, massage may be useful; otherwise there is no necessity for this treatment. Whenever required, massage should if possible be given by an experienced masseuse. If this is out of the question and the patient must rely upon one of her friends, it should be understood that "general massage" is needed; in other words, one part of the body after another should be gone over systematically. With an inexperienced masseuse, however, it will be safer not to massage the abdomen, since awkward, vigorous, or prolonged manipulations in that locality may provoke painful uterine contractions. Rubbing the breasts also can do no good; on the contrary, it may do harm by bruising them.

The best time of day to have massage is in the morning, at least an hour after breakfast. The duration of the treatment will depend upon the patient; it should always cease as soon as she begins to feel tired. After one has become accustomed to it, massage may generally be continued for an hour. The room in which it is given should be cool, and after the treatment has been completed the patient should be wrapped warmly and left undisturbed for half an hour.

Gymnastics, like massage, are useless to those who can enjoy outdoor exercise. Walking more perfectly strengthens the muscles which take part in the act of birth than any system of "home calisthenics" that has been suggested. In some conditions which make walking inadvisable the use of calisthenics will be helpful. These exercises generally consist in breathing movements and in movements of the extremities, especially the legs, which bring into play the same abdominal muscles that are used at the time of delivery. A detailed description of the exercises is here purposely omitted, since gymnastics should not be used unless advised by a physician, who should watch their effect and thus be guided as to whether the patient should continue them.

THE INFLUENCE OF WORK UPON PREGNANCY.--No single influence is more unfavorable to comfort and health during pregnancy than is idleness, so that every prospective should occupy herself with congenial work and fitting diversions. The kind of occupation makes no essential difference, so long as it does not overtire either the body or the mind. Since most women are absorbed in the affairs of the home, it may be well to begin by saying that the existence of pregnancy by no means requires the abandonment of domestic duties. On the contrary, when it is convenient, the prospective mother should have a share in the housework. She should not undertake everything that is to be done about the house, for no matter how small the household there are certain duties too laborious for her to attempt; these will be easily recognized and turned over to someone else. Even with regard to those tasks which lie within her strength she should use a little forethought to prevent unnecessary steps.

All kinds of violent exertion should be avoided--a rule which at once excludes sweeping, scrubbing, laundry work, lifting anything that is heavy, and going up and down stairs hurriedly or frequently. The use of a sewing machine is also emphatically forbidden. Treadle work is known to be one cause of swollen feet, of varicose veins, and of aches and pains in the legs or the abdomen. If a prospective mother has to do her own sewing, the machine should be fitted with a hand attachment or motor. Except for the possibility of straining the eyes, there is no objection to sewing by hand.

Besides the activities that should be excluded because they may be harmful, every housekeeper will find enough to keep her busy. It is generally not a small task to suggest what others shall do and to see that orders are properly carried out; consequently those who take no part in the actual work may retain an absorbing interest in their domestic affairs by directing them. Such direction, indeed, should, toward the end of pregnancy, constitute the mother's sole participation in the housework.

In a general way the amount and the kind of work that a woman may be permitted to undertake during pregnancy depend upon what she has been used to. It is not unlikely that anyone who is unaccustomed to manual labor may injure her health and cause the pregnancy to end prematurely if she undertakes hard work. On the other hand, women of the working classes sometimes continue at their occupations to the natural end of pregnancy without harmful consequences. It is undeniable, however, that among this class miscarriages are more frequent than among the well-to-do. Furthermore, the average birth- weight of mature infants whose mothers have remained at work during the last three months of pregnancy is ten per cent. less than the average birth-weight of infants among the leisure class. This matter of the baby's weight is not always serious in itself, but indicates in the case of working women who are pregnant the existence of a strain that sometimes leads to serious accidents.

The employment of women during pregnancy and immediately thereafter is regulated by law in many countries. For example, the laws of Holland, Belgium, England, Portugal, and Austria prohibit the employment of women in factories during the last four weeks of pregnancy or the four weeks following childbirth. Such employment is unlawful in Switzerland for two weeks before and six weeks after childbirth. There is no legal regulation of the employment of pregnant women in either Germany or Norway, but the laws of both countries forbid them to return to work until six weeks after they have been delivered. Among civilized nations Turkey, Russia, Spain, Italy, France, and the United States make no attempt to regulate employment either before or after childbirth.

Of course there are strong sentimental reasons for relieving prospective mothers of the necessity of earning a living, but there are also excellent hygienic reasons against many kinds of employment. For example, it should be unlawful to employ them in chemical industries where, owing to their condition, they are especially liable to be injured by the materials which they handle. Jacobi states that the worst occupation for pregnant women is working with metals, in particular lead; more than half of them suffer miscarriage or premature confinement. Furthermore, the health of the child may be endangered if the prospective mother does hard work of any kind. This is true chiefly because she does not have appropriate intervals of relaxation, for it is a firmly established principle that a prospective mother must be free to rest the moment she begins to feel tired. The least, therefore, that can be done to better prevalent conditions among women who must work during pregnancy is to require by law a reduction in the number of their working hours, and to protect them from the necessity of earning a living for two months after they have been delivered.

RELAXATION AND REST.--During the early months of pregnancy many women complain that they feel enervated, and tire quickly even when they do things which were formerly done with ease; this experience is so common that it can scarcely be considered other than natural. Curiously enough this is also the period during which the attachment of the ovum to the womb is relatively insecure, and therefore the inclination to be quiet is justified by the prevailing anatomical conditions. No prospective mother should struggle against the inclination to rest; she should yield to it in spite of the advice to the contrary which older women are apt to give. Furthermore, it is especially important about the time when a menstrual period would ordinarily be expected to be guided by this impulse not to be active, since overexertion then, more than at other times, is apt to be followed by miscarriage. Except in rare cases the observance of this precaution is less urgent after the fourth month, when the ovum has become more securely attached to the womb. But again, toward the end of pregnancy the development of the mother's body necessitates a comparatively large amount of rest; patients who continue to exert themselves may expect to suffer from shortness of breath and a number of other annoyances.

In order to save needless steps and to avoid confusion and worry, it is always helpful to map out beforehand what must be done in the course of the day. Ideally, such a schedule should set apart intervals for relaxation and rest. In the morning, for example, while the housework is in progress, it is important to stop occasionally, if only for a few moments, and lie down on a couch. After the midday meal it is advisable to undress and go to bed. Even though one does not fall asleep, an hour or two of complete relaxation will be beneficial. A nap in the afternoon does not interfere with sleeping at night provided plenty of exercise has been taken during the day. In this way walking in the late afternoon or early evening helps to secure a good night's rest.

During the first six or seven months, pregnancy, in itself, does not cause sleeplessness, but later, as a natural result of the enlargement of the womb, there are several disagreeable symptoms which may cause broken rest at night. In the later months the weight of the womb requires women to sleep on the side, and for some of them this position is awkward at first. Frequently the pressure makes it necessary to get up several times during the night to empty the bladder. In a few cases also the compression of the chest interferes somewhat with breathing. When insomnia is due to the pressure of the womb against neighboring parts of the body, it can be partially counteracted by getting into a comfortable position; but it is also necessary to have the surroundings as conducive to sleep as possible. Thus anyone will be much more likely to rest well if the bed-room is large and well ventilated, if the mattress is comfortable, and if the coverings are warm without being heavy. Finally, not the least important detail is to occupy a single bed, so that it is possible to turn over without fear of disturbing someone else.

In most instances, however, the inability to sleep during pregnancy-- and indeed at any time--is due to a faulty frame of mind. With reference to the average man or woman, in his very helpful book "Why Worry," Walton says, "it is futile to expect that a fretful, impatient, and overanxious frame of mind, continuing through the day and every day, will be suddenly replaced at night by the placid and comfortable mental state which shall insure a restful sleep." Like everyone else, the prospective mother must stop thinking when she retires, otherwise the blood will not be diverted from the brain as it must be to fall asleep. To aid in bringing about this condition a number of expedients may be employed. For example, a warm bath, warm sheets, or a hot-water bottle placed against the feet all help to draw the blood from the brain to other parts of the body. Similarly, a warm glass of milk or a small portion of easily digestible solid food taken just before retiring will help to make one drowsy; on the other hand, over-eating at the evening meal or later is not an infrequent cause of wakefulness.

The use of narcotics is rarely necessary in the early months of pregnancy, and the simple measures just mentioned will also generally be found sufficient in the later months. But these procedures, or any other except the use of strong drugs, will be ineffective unless the individual knows how to get into the proper state of mind. This means not only that she must be able to banish worries, regrets, and forebodings; she must also have acquired confidence in whatever method she employs. She must convince herself that she can sleep, or at least that it makes no difference if she cannot. This independent spirit, which is very essential, can be confidently assumed, for if she does not sleep well it can be made up during the next day or at least the next night. Having adopted this attitude, and having assumed a comfortable position, which should be retained as long as possible, the attention should be concentrated upon the thought, "I am getting sleepy, I am going to sleep." Under these circumstances she can hypnotize herself and "produce the desired result more often than by watching the proverbial sheep follow one another over the wall."

IS TRAVELING HARMFUL?--Traveling has been made so easy and alluring that nowadays long journeys are undertaken with scarcely more concern than was once felt when the people of neighboring towns exchanged visits. Thus modern facilities have introduced a new factor into the problem of the way to live during pregnancy. It is a well-known fact that traveling is sometimes attended with risk to the prospective mother, though the danger is exaggerated in the popular estimation. For this the newspapers are chiefly to blame. They inform the public of the cases in which embarrassing situations have arisen, but there is no record of the thousands of pregnant women who travel without any mishap.

What the effect of traveling is likely to be is very difficult to predict under any circumstances, and the question cannot be answered at all unless the specific conditions presented by each case are taken into account. In a general way the points to be considered are the vigor of the patient, the period of pregnancy at which she has arrived, and the character of the journey she wishes to undertake. Prudent women will never attempt to decide this question for themselves, but will always obtain professional advice. The disapproval of the physician, no doubt, will sometimes cause keen disappointment; but conservative advice is the best and should always be followed.

To be on the safe side a prospective mother who has previously had a miscarriage should not travel at any time during pregnancy; others are not obliged to follow this stringent rule except during the first sixteen and the last four weeks of pregnancy. In the former period there is some danger of miscarriage because traveling may cause separation of the relatively loose attachment of the ovum. In the latter period the muscle-fibers of the womb are usually irritable and therefore the rolling of a ship or the jolting of a car may set up painful contractions which in some instances expel the fetus. Generally there is the least risk of accident between the eighteenth and the thirty-second weeks, though patients should be careful even during this interval not to travel at the time when a menstrual period would ordinarily be expected.

The length of the journey and the ease with which it can be made are also important features to be considered. Obviously there will be less danger of mishap from a short trip than from a long one; if possible, therefore, long journeys by rail should be broken so as to afford opportunity for rest. Railroad trips which do not exceed two or three hours are generally not so fatiguing that they must be prohibited, provided the individual is perfectly well. Traveling by boat is less tiresome than traveling by rail and, if equally convenient, the boat should be given the preference. Long automobile tours are attended with considerable risk of miscarriage and, therefore, are forbidden.

MENTAL DIVERSION.--As a rule good health prevails throughout pregnancy; it would be enjoyed even more frequently if many prospective mothers did not think so much about the fact that they are pregnant. For this deplorable self-consciousness the spirit of the age is in part to blame; there never was a time, in all probability, when people took such a keen interest in all matters pertaining to health. It is also true, however, that fuller instruction is needed now because the temptations to depart from a regular, temperate way of living have notably increased.

At all events the point has now been reached where the average man or woman knows something of anatomy, physiology, and the laws of hygiene. Such knowledge should be helpful, and generally is, but if it causes anyone to think incessantly about the workings of the body, to that person it is detrimental. We all know such individuals. They are made miserable because they scrutinize functions, like the beating of the heart, that go on automatically and should be left unobserved, or they minutely analyze their feelings and misinterpret normal sensations as the evidence of disease.

The tendency to be introspective is especially pronounced in women who are pregnant, and this is readily explained by the reciprocal relations between the mind and the body. If the prospective mother correctly interpreted the changes which occur in her body, as well as the sensations for which these changes are responsible, she would escape the uneasiness of mind that causes many sorts of discomfort. It is unfortunately true, however, that her lack of familiarity with the facts about pregnancy and her belief in unfounded traditions frequently lead to the misinterpretation of natural conditions. An anxious frame of mind also causes real ailments to assume an importance out of all proportion to their actual significance.

Patients who have followed my advice to place themselves in the care of a physician as soon as they clearly recognize the existence of pregnancy will receive his assistance in properly estimating the significance of what they notice. This service is by no means the least the obstetrician renders his patients. His opinion should always be sought when symptoms are not understood; but it is not unusual for patients to bring to the doctor's attention many complaints that would pass unnoticed if they taught themselves to restrain the imagination, to refrain from pessimistic reflections, and to divert their thoughts from themselves to outside affairs.

Generally it is during the early months of pregnancy that patients are most likely to be self-centered, and consequently suffer from many annoyances that either proceed from or are exaggerated by this faulty frame of mind. During this period a prospective mother is not fully aware of the meaning of pregnancy. Toward the twentieth week, however, she perceives the movements of the child and her thoughts are turned to it instinctively. About this time many of the discomforts of pregnancy disappear and there ensues a period of unusually good health. Perhaps it would be going too far to give this more wholesome altruistic mental attitude the entire credit for the relatively better health of the second half of pregnancy, but without doubt it is a most important factor.

Such then is the influence of the mind over the body that anyone who wishes to cultivate good health must correct the faulty habit of always thinking of herself. The most suitable form of diversion will depend upon personal taste. Domestic duties absorb the attention of most prospective mothers, but domestic duties should not occupy them exclusively. Outdoor recreation is necessary and serves the double purpose of strengthening mind and body. Public amusements should also be patronized; no prospective mother has the right to sacrifice herself to pride. Music, the various arts, a systematic course of reading, the acquisition of a foreign language--all these are commendable forms of diversion, and others will occur to anyone. Obviously the avocation will be most happily chosen if it directs the attention into channels likely to lead to the greatest pleasure.

CHAPTER VII

THE AILMENTS OF PREGNANCY

Nausea and Vomiting--Heartburn--Flatulence--Defective Teeth--Pressure Symptoms: Swelling of the Feet; Varicose Veins; Hemorrhoids; Shortness of Breath--Leucorrhea--Toxemias.

Most of the ailments to which prospective mothers are liable are merely the natural manifestations of pregnancy, exaggerated to such an extent as to cause inconvenience and discomfort. In the early months, for example, persistent nausea and vomiting may become the source of great annoyance, and later the pressure of the womb against neighboring structures may cause a variety of symptoms. It does not follow, however, that any of these ailments will necessarily appear. On the contrary, many women are more healthy during pregnancy than at any other time.

Occasionally illness is charged to pregnancy with which in reality pregnancy has nothing to do. While awaiting the birth of a child, just as at other times, women may suffer from coughs or colds, from aches or pains, from malaria, pneumonia, typhoid fever, or in fact from any disease. It is evident that such complications are accidental; and, though pregnancy confers no immunity against them, it does not, on the other hand, render women more susceptible to all kinds of ailment.

And yet there are diseases for which pregnancy is directly responsible. These are, to a very large extent, preventable; and, though they occur rarely, precautions for their prevention should be taken in every case of pregnancy. By far the most important members of this group are the toxemias of pregnancy. These, as will be explained later, cause symptoms which the patient herself may recognize, and her physician may often detect their presence still earlier by alterations in the composition of the urine. For this reason routine examination of the urine during pregnancy is a means of prevention indispensable for safeguarding the health of the prospective mother.

A number of ailments of which prospective mothers may complain do not require treatment with medicine. This, however, will not be taken to imply that there is no need to consult a physician. On the contrary, and it cannot be emphasized too strongly, the prospective mother should seek professional service whenever there is anything about her condition she does not understand. Sometimes, when she thus consults the physician, he will explain to her that what she has noticed is merely one of the natural manifestations of pregnancy and that she can have no control over it; at other times he will suggest changes in her mode of life which will very likely afford her relief. The frequency with which physicians find that ailments may be corrected by the adoption of hygienic measures indicates that such ailments are more often due to ignorance or carelessness than to the existence of disease.

NAUSEA AND VOMITING.--We have already learned that nausea, especially in the morning on rising from bed, frequently corroborates the suspicion of a woman that she has become pregnant. So commonly, indeed, is this symptom expected that most women take no account of it other than as an evidence that they have conceived, and consequently do not complain of it. A few who have heard the old adage, "a sick pregnancy means a safe one," which incidentally is not correct, actually accept nausea as a favorable sign. In other cases the nausea is not to be dismissed so lightly; and a relatively small group of patients suffer from persistent vomiting. When prospective mothers are questioned systematically, it appears that at least one- half and perhaps two-thirds of them experience more or less discomfort from sick stomach. Generally this begins shortly after a menstrual period has been missed and ceases six or eight weeks later; it persists occasionally until the movements of the child have been perceived.

Nausea and vomiting are limited, in the vast majority of cases, to the early morning, but some patients are annoyed only after meals, and a few at irregular intervals during the day. The fact that the attacks do not always appear at the same time, and that they differ in severity, indicates that different causes may be concerned in their production. And it is true that there are several kinds of vomiting that occur during pregnancy, although the classification interests only physicians. The laity, however, should understand that the treatment of any given case will vary according to the class to which it belongs, and therefore the occurrence of troublesome vomiting should be promptly reported to the physician.

Most frequently it will be found that there is nothing serious the matter. The vomiting ceases or, at least, it becomes less troublesome as soon as the diet has been more carefully arranged, constipation has been corrected, or other hygienic details, such as outdoor recreation and mental diversion, have received the attention requisite for good health. In a much smaller group of cases the restoration of the womb to a proper position or the treatment of some other local condition, which can generally be remedied without difficulty, is all that is necessary. But finally, in extremely rare instances, the vomiting of pregnancy is due to a definite disease whose existence may be recognized by special methods of analyzing the urine. In any case, if the physician is given an opportunity to make the necessary observations and thus determine the variety of the vomiting, no time will be lost in beginning effective treatment. In an overwhelming majority of the cases, as I have said, nothing serious will be found; and then the control of the vomiting will lie within the power of the patient herself.

Since nausea is usually experienced in the morning on rising from the recumbent to the upright posture, measures to prevent an attack should be begun even before the patient raises her head from the pillow. In the first place something to eat should be taken as soon as she awakens. The most satisfactory results follow eating two or three pieces of crisp toast or a Bent's cracker (sold by grocers), either of which should be thoroughly chewed and swallowed without taking anything to drink. Good results are also obtained, though less uniformly, from eating other food, such as fruit, oatmeal, or eggs. The benefit secured from this procedure is explained, perhaps, by the activity of the digestive organs and the effect of that activity upon the circulation of the blood. The food eaten before rising is not intended to take the place of breakfast, which ordinarily will be eaten later. Furthermore, it is essential to remain in bed until half an hour after the food was taken; and not to rise then unless perfectly comfortable. Anyone who is inclined to be nauseated should get up slowly and dress leisurely, sitting down as much as possible while putting on the clothes. If breakfast is not desired at once, it should not be forced, but some food should be eaten between early morning and noon.

It is an exceedingly good rule to bend every effort toward escaping the initial attack of nausea, for in this way one soon gains confidence, and overcomes the depressing habit of being continually on the watch for the symptom, lest she be taken unawares. Exceptionally, however, patients feel more comfortable if they vomit in the morning; this may be helpful, for example, if a large meal has been eaten just before retiring the previous night.

Next to morning sickness in point of frequency comes the disposition to be nauseated about meal time. Those who vomit after the meal is finished are frequently inclined to eat soon again; and there is no reason why they should not. Sick stomach after meals may be due to several causes, such as eating hurriedly, eating too much, or selecting food that is difficult to digest. If a meal is bolted the stomach may be overloaded before the appetite is appeased; and consequently those who eat too much are fortunate when the stomach rejects the excess. Eating slowly and masticating the food thoroughly, we know, is the proper way to insure taking no more than is needed.

One of the most valuable precautions against persistent nausea consists in taking small amounts of food five or six times during the day. Directions regarding the frequency of meals and the choice of food have been given in Chapter IV, to which the reader may refer. It may be repeated, however, that a prospective mother should naturally avoid anything which she knows is likely not to agree with her. On the other hand, she is almost certain not to be nauseated by any article of food for which she has an appetite.

Lying down for a short while after meals frequently serves to prevent an attack of vomiting. It is a good rule, furthermore, at whatever time of day the sensation of nausea may occur, to lie down immediately. An ice bag or cloths wrung out of cold water, if applied to the abdomen, often give relief; warm applications occasionally serve the same purpose better. Some patients prevent nausea by constantly wearing a flannel bandage about the abdomen.

Many instances of the vomiting of pregnancy cannot be explained by errors in diet, for the attacks come on repeatedly whether the stomach contains food or not. Under these circumstances mental influences frequently have to be reckoned with. Indeed, in most cases of vomiting of pregnancy dietetic and other hygienic measures are of no avail unless the patient learns to divert her attention from troublesome thoughts.

That the brain can exert an influence over the stomach is a fact well substantiated both by physiological experiment and by medical observation. In all probability there is a definite spot in the brain, called the "vomiting center," the irritation of which causes retching and the upheaval of the contents of the stomach. As this nervous mechanism is possessed by everyone, it is not called into existence by the advent of pregnancy. Nevertheless, it seems likely that pregnancy renders it more sensitive, and it is certain that pregnancy establishes new means by which the center may be stimulated. This admission does not imply, however, that the prospective mother must submit to inevitable discomfort, for she can and should muster the strength to resist it.

Time and again an unhappy frame of mind exaggerates or prolongs the vomiting of pregnancy. Thus, disappointment, anxiety, grief, fright, and other types of mental uneasiness not only magnify the discomfort but sometimes are its sole cause. The curious cases in which the husband suffers from nausea while his wife is pregnant are explained by mental influences. As a result of the same kind of influence, women who imagine themselves to be pregnant often suffer from violent vomiting, which ceases as soon as they discover their error. On the other hand, women who for several months remain ignorant of the fact that they are pregnant rarely suffer from sick stomach.

Any kind of worry may be and often is the direct cause of the vomiting of pregnancy, though patients are often unwilling to confess it; and occasionally do not seem to know what it is that troubles them. In any event, having received the assurance of her physician that there is nothing serious the matter, the prospective mother who is annoyed by nausea should make every effort not to become self- centered. She should have congenial companionship and should interest herself in pursuits outside of, as well as within, her home. Of all the measures that may be employed to overcome this manifestation of pregnancy the most fundamental and essential is mental diversion.

HEARTBURN.--Obviously, it would not be fair to consider indigestion as one of the ailments peculiar to pregnancy, for anyone is liable to suffer from indigestion. Yet dyspeptic symptoms, more especially heartburn and flatulence, occur so frequently at this time that something should be said regarding their causation and treatment.

A burning sensation rising from the stomach into the throat, familiarly called heartburn, is generally due to an overabundant secretion of hydrochloric acid, which is, as we have learned, a normal constituent of the gastric juice. Of late, the conditions which influence its secretion have been the subject of laboratory investigation, which has disclosed, among other interesting facts, the way to prevent heartburn. These experiments have taught that the introduction of fat into the stomach shortly before a meal decreases the amount of acid secreted during digestion. Consequently, anyone who is troubled by heartburn and wishes to avoid it _should take a tablespoonful of olive oil, a cup of cream, or a glass of rich milk fifteen or twenty minutes before meal-time_.

On the other hand, fatty food eaten with the meals prolongs the stay of food in the stomach and causes an increase in the secretion of hydrochloric acid. An excess of the acid, as we have just learned, is favorable to the development of heartburn. Therefore, as a further precaution against this source of discomfort, it is advisable not to use a large amount of butter or of salad oil, and to refrain from fried food, rich desserts, or any other article of diet known to contain a relatively large amount of fat.

Once it has developed, heartburn will be aggravated by taking cream or olive oil. The most rational curative measures then consist in diluting the acid by drinking a couple of glasses of water and in counteracting (neutralizing) the acid by taking a teaspoonful of baking soda (bicarbonate of soda) or a tablespoonful of limewater; and, if necessary, either of these doses may be repeated. Patients often adopt the very sensible habit of carrying with them a block of magnesium carbonate, which they nibble whenever the symptom appears.

FLATULENCE.--The distention of stomach and intestines with gas, technically called flatulence, may be associated with heartburn or appear independently. The gas arises from the action of bacteria upon the food. There can be little doubt that flatulence occurs so regularly during pregnancy because the pressure of the enlarged womb prevents the contents of the intestine from moving along as rapidly as they have done previously.

To be relieved from this source of discomfort, it is necessary, in the first place, that the bowels should be regularly evacuated; very often nothing further is required than to overcome the habit of constipation. Occasionally, however, the diet must be arranged so as to exclude food which is likely to form gas. For example, parsnips, beans, corn, fried food, candy, cake, and sweet desserts, all of which are known to cause flatulence, should be avoided; in aggravated cases the allowance of starchy food of every kind should be cut down to small portions.

Since the production of gas in the intestine is due to the action of bacteria sometimes relief from flatulence is secured only after the administration of intestinal antiseptics. Drugs, however, will be prescribed by the physician, and will not be employed until the simpler hygienic measures have failed. Similarly, the physician should decide whether it is advisable for the patient to drink milk inoculated with harmless bacteria (The Bulgarian Bacillus) which has lately been placed on the market. The bacteria thus administered in the milk are antagonistic to the intestinal bacteria that produce gas, and consequently have been recommended for the treatment of flatulence. If this commercial product cannot be conveniently obtained, one may use instead tablets containing the bacteria, which can be supplied by druggists.

DEFECTIVE TEETH.--Unless suitable precautions are observed, the digestive disturbances of pregnancy have a tendency to injure the teeth. The regurgitation of the acid contents of the stomach, for example, may cause cavities to develop or may enlarge those that already exist. In all probability the damage done in this way--and not the removal of lime from the teeth for the formation of the child's skeleton, as some have thought--is responsible for the origin of the saying that "every child costs a tooth." This notion is of course absurd, yet it is quite true that toothache and the decay or loosening of the teeth are not infrequently associated with pregnancy. On this account, throughout the period of pregnancy particular care should be given the teeth.

One of the very first duties of a prospective mother, after she knows that conception has taken place, is to visit her dentist. This step is very important as a means of insuring the teeth against such harmful influence as pregnancy may have upon them. If the dentist finds the teeth in poor condition, the patient should consent to have them treated immediately. That this is the reasonable course seems sufficiently obvious, yet the majority of women have been slow to adopt such a view.

For a long time dental work of every description was incorrectly believed to have an untoward effect upon the development of the child; and the extraction of a tooth, it was thought, would surely be followed by miscarriage. Although the extraction of teeth is not frequently undertaken nowadays, I have known several prospective mothers who required the operation, and who had it performed without experiencing a single untoward symptom. Very naturally dental work should be restricted during pregnancy to that which is absolutely necessary, and temporary fillings generally suffice; but whatever is needed should be done without delay.

Brushing the teeth after meals and removing particles of food that may have been caught between them--important enough at all times--are of even greater importance during pregnancy. If the gums are sore and the teeth show a tendency to loosen, the best tooth-paste is one containing potassium chlorate.

An alkaline mouth-wash should be used several times a day; after an attack of vomiting it is always advisable to rinse the mouth with such a solution. As a wash either lime water or milk of magnesia, or a solution of bicarbonate of soda may be used; they are equally good. Lime water may be prepared at home inexpensively in the following way: Place a teacupful of builders' lime in a large bowl and add two quarts of water; thoroughly mix and allow to settle. Pour off and throw the water away, since it often contains impurities. Add two quarts of water again and allow the mixture to stand three or four hours, stirring occasionally. Strain through a piece of muslin into bottles and keep well corked. One tablespoonful of this solution should be added to a glass of water to obtain the proper strength for a mouth-wash.

PRESSURE SYMPTOMS.--Because human beings walk erect, and not on all fours, they are liable to suffer from various ailments of pregnancy that quadrupeds escape. Thus the upright posture is the chief factor, at least, in causing such complaints as swollen feet, varicose veins, hemorrhoids, and cramps in the legs. The attention of patients should be called to the source of these troubles, for in most instances they can be prevented by forethought and prudence.

During the last two or three months of pregnancy every prospective mother should carefully avoid being too much on her feet; she should lie down, as has already been emphasized, at regular times of day and frequently sit down to rest. Proper support for the abdomen, such as is afforded by a correct corset or a maternity supporter, lifts the pregnant uterus, and to a notable extent relieves of pressure the structures beneath it. On the other hand, incorrectly made corsets, the use of circular garters, and running a sewing machine by foot- power all aggravate the pressure symptoms of pregnancy.

Swelling of the Feet.--So long as the swelling is confined to the feet and legs it does not mean that there is trouble with the kidneys; the swelling is satisfactorily explained by the pressure of the enlarged uterus upon the veins which pass through the lower part of the abdomen and conduct the blood from the legs on its way back to the heart. The womb is rarely heavy enough during the first half of pregnancy to interfere with the flow of blood through these vessels, but in the last few months such interference is very common.

Generally the limbs are equally affected, yet occasionally the swelling is more marked on one side or the other. The characteristic changes begin in the feet. The skin covering the back of the foot becomes tense and has a waxen appearance; it is easily indented, bearing for a moment the imprint of anything that is pressed against it. Often the swelling extends no higher than the ankles, but it may involve the calves, the thighs, or even the vulva, which is the region between the thighs.

If the swelling remains slight, no attention need be paid to it. But if it becomes extensive or painful, nothing will give relief except going to bed.

Patients observe for themselves that the swelling lessens during the night, and from this usually learn that the proper treatment is rest. When it is absolutely impossible to remain in bed long enough for the swelling to disappear, the next best plan is to accept every opportunity, during the day, to sit down and prop up the feet.

Varicose Veins.--The distention of the surface veins of the legs, the condition known as varicose veins, is not a peculiarity of pregnancy. Anyone who must be on his feet a great deal is liable to suffer from this ailment. It is true, nevertheless, that pregnancy increases the likelihood of the development of varicose veins. The walls of the vessel are generally able to withstand whatever strain is placed upon them during the first pregnancy, and usually the varicosed condition does not develop until after there have been several pregnancies.

As a rule, both legs are similarly affected, but if only one, it is more likely to be the right. This is explained by the fact that the position of the child within the womb is ordinarily such as to cause greater pressure on the vessels of the right side. For the same reason when the legs are unequally affected, generally the veins of the right side are the larger. In any case, however, the birth of the child removes the source of the interference, and during the lying-in period, provided that the patient remains quiet for a sufficient length of time, the vessels regain their normal caliber. Once they have been distended, however, the veins remain more susceptible to engorgement. Consequently, in order not to increase the strain these vessels naturally bear during the latter months of pregnancy, the precautions just mentioned for the avoidance of all the pressure symptoms should be strictly observed. Upon the first intimation that the veins are becoming dilated, a patient should be unusually careful to keep off her feet all that she can. Only in extreme cases will it be compulsory to go to bed. But, if the veins are large and painful, she should stay in bed until material improvement has taken place. Subsequently she should wear a flannel bandage, snugly applied, about the leg from the toes to a point somewhat above the knee; the bandage should extend higher whenever the veins of the thigh also are dilated. In putting on the bandage the heel may be left uncovered; after leaving the foot a turn of the bandage will be taken around the ankle and thence applied upward. A flannel bandage may be easily made at home. Bias strips are cut about three inches in width and sewed together end to end so that the joining will lie flat. Unless the bandage must extend far above the knee, eight yards will be a sufficient length.

Elastic stockings, which may be purchased from a druggist, serve the same purpose as the bandage, but are very much less durable. Even if worn during the day they should be taken off at night; and when protection of the veins is required after going to bed, the bandage is the most sanitary way of securing it.

The danger that one of the vessels will break may be disregarded, if they are constantly protected by the measures that have been mentioned. In the event of accident, however, make firm pressure over the bleeding point with a freshly laundered handkerchief, and apply an ice bag outside the dressing until the doctor arrives.

Hemorrhoids.--Hemorrhoids are caused in the same way as varicose veins of the legs. The two conditions differ merely in point of location; but hemorrhoids, on account of their location, are much more exposed to irritation.

Although the development of hemorrhoids cannot always be prevented, it is a well-known fact that constipation renders the chance of their appearance much greater. In a measure, therefore, regular, daily evacuation of the bowels serves to prevent the ailment, and also to cure it, once it has developed. But walking and even standing aggravate hemorrhoids. The recumbent posture, as might be expected, is of itself frequently enough to give relief. It is much more likely to do so, however, if the hips are elevated by placing a pillow under them.

In severe cases it is helpful to restrict the diet for a few days until the congestion and acute suffering have subsided. If the hemorrhoids protrude, they should be replaced (which the patient may generally do for herself), and an ice bag should be applied to the seat of pain. Various ointments and suppositories of different composition are valuable in the treatment of this ailment, but, as not all cases are relieved by the same medicine, a physician should be consulted to learn what is most suitable in any given instance.

Hemorrhoids often grow progressively worse as pregnancy advances, and are frequently aggravated immediately after the birth of the child; but they generally disappear within a few weeks. Whenever a natural cure is not thus effected, it may become necessary to resort to surgical treatment. Operative procedures, however, should not be undertaken during pregnancy, since the condition is likely to reappear before the child is born.

Cramps in the Legs.--There are nerves as well as blood vessels that the pregnant uterus may press upon, and pressure of this kind may cause pain. At times the pain is definitely localized at the point where the nerve is pressed upon; under these circumstances the discomfort is felt in the lower part of the back. On the other hand, the pain may be referred to the point where the nerve ends. In this way is explained not only pain in the leg but also those sensations of numbness and tingling which prospective mothers not infrequently complain of. The presence of these pressure symptoms is usually limited to the last few weeks of pregnancy. They often begin about the time the child's head enters the bony canal through which it is ultimately born; engagement of the head, as this is called, occurs simultaneously with the dropping of the waist-line, that is, about two or three weeks before delivery. From the time the head is engaged all the pressure symptoms become somewhat more intense.

From the very nature of their causation, it is clear that cramps in the legs are difficult to treat. The recumbent posture lessens the discomfort, and, if in addition the hips are elevated, absolute comfort will occasionally be secured. Whether or not the administration of medicine is advisable must be determined by the physician who has the opportunity to see the patient. The birth of the child, of course, removes the cause of the pressure and permanently relieves this discomfort.

Shortness of Breath.--Besides the ailments caused by the downward pressure of the pregnant uterus, there are also symptoms due to its upward growth. Thus shortness of breath is regularly noted toward the end of pregnancy, and, as has already been mentioned, it is one of the reasons for exercising leisurely.

Unlike the other pressure symptoms, shortness of breath is ordinarily aggravated by the recumbent posture, for lying flat on the back increases the compression of the chest. At night, which is frequently the time when difficulty in breathing is most pronounced, the patient may, if necessary, sleep propped up in bed. For this purpose an appliance called a back-rest may be used, but an extra pillow under the head and shoulders is usually sufficient.

LEUCORRHEA.--The meaning of the white discharge from the vagina known as leucorrhea is variable: at times it indicates the existence of an ailment requiring treatment, and at other times it does not. To be on the safe side, therefore, anyone who is troubled by leucorrhea should obtain her physician's opinion as to its significance.

Normally, as we learned in Chapter V, there is an increase in the vaginal secretion during pregnancy; but this fact is rarely noticeable until the latter months. Usually it is pronounced only during the last few weeks. At that time, owing to its antiseptic qualities, this pale white fluid should not be disturbed by the use of douches. In the early months of pregnancy, however, leucorrhea may cause such inconvenience as to demand medical treatment.

While itching is the most disagreeable effect of such a vaginal discharge, it should be known that itching is not always due to leucorrhea. Thus it may be caused by a highly concentrated urine, and in that event will be relieved by drinking a larger amount of water; or it may be due to the presence of unusual constituents in the urine. Skin diseases also cause itching; and light haired people, since they have more delicate skins that brunettes, are especially susceptible to these ailments. To such skin affections soap and water may be very irritating; so that when they exist it is often advisable to cleanse the parts with olive oil. In other cases, ointments are required and will be prescribed by the physician.

Itching of the skin over the extremities or over the whole body, it is clear, cannot be attributed to leucorrhea, but in these very rare cases the irritation would seem to be caused by some waste product which is being eliminated through the sweat glands. We do not know what the substance is, but, as the symptom appears so seldom, it must be due to an unusual kind of waste product or else to one whose elimination normally occurs through other channels. The affection of the skin thus brought about is really a very mild kind of poisoning, and since the offending substance arises in the body of the patient herself the condition is called an autointoxication. Effective treatment consists in drinking water freely and taking a cathartic, for the one stimulates the kidneys and the other the bowels to assist in getting rid of the cause of the trouble.

TOXEMIAS.--In order to understand what are known as the toxemias of pregnancy, we must remember that the nutrition of our bodies involves three separate and distinct sets of processes. What we eat is, in the first place, digested and absorbed into the body; secondly, the products of digestion are utilized by the tissues; and, finally, the waste material is thrown off from the body. Any one of these processes may be carried out in a way that is not consistent with health. Most of us realize that disturbances may occur in the course of digestion, and we are also aware that the excretory organs occasionally fail to do their work in a satisfactory way. But what laymen, perhaps, do not appreciate is that the intermediary steps-- between the time when the food is absorbed and the time when the waste material is finally eliminated--may not be taken precisely as health requires. Of course, any person may be the subject of one or another of these nutritional disorders, but unquestionably such disorders are somewhat more frequent during pregnancy than at other times. Nor is this difficult to understand, for the nutritional processes of two beings are here linked together. They generally proceed harmoniously, but if they do not there results an autointoxication of the mother which is called a toxemia.

Such toxemias, with extremely rare exceptions, do not occur in the early months, but are associated with the period of the active growth of the fetus, namely, the second half of pregnancy. For this reason, and for some others which do not concern us here, it seems probable that the nutritional processes of the child are primarily responsible for these ailments. This view, however, must be somewhat modified, for experience has clearly taught that the efficiency with which the maternal excretory organs do their work has a great deal to do with the effect that the fetal waste products have upon the mother. On this account she has been urged to pay attention to personal hygiene. It is also necessary, however, that she should become acquainted with the symptoms which give warning that the excretory organs are acting imperfectly.

Autointoxication can almost always be prevented. The means of prevention are neither mysterious nor difficult to carry out; they lie within the power of every prospective mother, for they consist merely of what has already been discussed, namely, the intelligent regulation of the diet, the care of the body, and a correct ordering of the daily life. To the chapters dealing with these subjects reference should be made and particular attention should be paid to what has been said concerning:

(1) Wearing suitably warm clothes, (2) Bathing regularly, (3) Taking a proper amount of exercise, (4) Drinking water liberally, (5) Avoiding an excessive quantity of meat, (6) Guarding against constipation.

At present the value of prevention in the treatment of the toxemias of pregnancy is so clearly recognized that charitable organizations employ nurses to visit women of the poorer classes during pregnancy in order to instruct them about the measures that I have just indicated. Remarkable results have already been obtained. In one clinic where this method has been adopted the frequency of all kinds of toxemia, I am told, has notably diminished, and serious types are not permitted to develop. Similar results should be obtained in private practice when patients place themselves under medical supervision at the beginning of pregnancy. Under these favorable circumstances symptoms of autointoxication probably occur not oftener than once in every hundred pregnancies, but nine out of ten of them, being promptly recognized, yield readily to relatively simple treatment.

The early detection of such complications depends largely upon the patient herself. As has been emphasized--and it cannot be said too frequently--she should not fail to submit, at appropriate intervals, a specimen of urine for examination. It is by such an examination generally that the development of a toxemia is first detected. Occasionally, however, significant signs will attract the patient's attention before there is any change in the urine. For that reason, it is important to notify the physician if any of the following symptoms appear:

(1) Serious vomiting. (2) Persistent headache. (3) Dizziness. (4) Puffiness about the face. (5) Blurring of vision, or the appearance of black spots before the eyes. (6) Neuralgic pains, especially in the pit of the stomach.

It must be clearly understood, however, that any of these symptoms may be present without indicating that a toxemia is developing. Nevertheless, they should be brought to the physician's attention without delay, and, at the same time, a specimen of urine should be given him for examination.

Although the kidneys are not responsible for all the toxemias of pregnancy, an analysis of the urine affords the most definite means of determining whether or not such a condition is present. When thus detected, prompt treatment will guarantee to the patient almost certain relief. On the other hand if, as usually happens, the analysis shows conclusively that there is nothing serious the matter, this reassurance fully justifies the trouble taken to secure it.

CHAPTER VIII

MISCARRIAGE

Frequency--Causes and Prevention--Habitual Miscarriage--Warning Symptoms--After-effects--Criminal Abortion--Therapeutic Abortion-- Premature Delivery.

We have learned that forty weeks are required for the full development of the human embryo, but this fact carries no assurance that pregnancy will last so long; in reality, it may end abruptly at any time. If growth is interrupted before the twenty-eighth week (the seventh lunar month), the infant will be too immature to live. Even when born alive, it will usually perish within a few hours, or a few days at most. Children born during the seventh month have occasionally survived; but the prevalent belief that they are more likely to do so than if born a month later is erroneous. That superstition originated at a time when great virtue was ascribed to numbers. Since seven was a sacred number, it was considered more auspicious to be born in the seventh month than in the eighth. Universal experience, however, teaches us that the likelihood of rearing a premature child is, by a rapidly increasing proportion, the greater for every week that it remains within the uterus. This is precisely what we should expect, for the period of its existence there measures the perfection of its development; and that, under ordinary conditions, determines how strong and hardy the child will be.

Although during the first six months the outlook for the infant will be equally unfavorable at whatever time pregnancy may be interrupted, physicians prefer to distinguish cases which terminate in the earlier part of this period from those which terminate in the latter part. For technical reasons, the sixteenth week represents a natural point of division. A birth which takes place before that time is called an abortion; one which takes place between the sixteenth and the twenty- eighth week is called a miscarriage. The anatomical reasons which justify such a distinction do not concern us here, and the matter deserves mention merely because the same terms are often employed in a very different sense by the laity. As most of us know, the interruption of pregnancy results sometimes from purely natural causes, and sometimes from the employment of artificial means. As a rule, persons who are unacquainted with medical terminology call a birth of the former kind a miscarriage, and reserve the term abortion for an interruption of pregnancy that is deliberately provoked. Physicians, however, make no such distinction. They use these words, as I have said, simply to indicate how far development has progressed before the termination of pregnancy. Since the term abortion is apt to carry with it the implication of a criminal act, confusion will be avoided if we agree for the time to depart from strictly medical usage and designate as miscarriage the spontaneous termination of pregnancy prior to the twenty-eighth week.

FREQUENCY.--Early interruption of pregnancy is extremely common. Some sociologists declare that it is becoming more and more frequent, and see in it a grave national danger. French statesmen attribute the alarming decline of the birth-rate in their country, in great part, to a rapid increase in the number of pregnancies which end prematurely. Reliable English and German statistics indicate that of the pregnancies which come under the observation of physicians approximately twenty per cent, end in miscarriage. In our own country, though extensive and complete data are not available, it is likely that the incidence is equally high.

The actual frequency of miscarriage is generally underestimated. Patients themselves often do not know what has really happened. When the accident occurs a few days after conception, bleeding may be its only evidence, which will almost certainly be misinterpreted as an irregularity of menstruation; and professional advice will not often be thought necessary. Moreover, in other cases in which the true situation is appreciated the patient does not feel sick enough to seek medical assistance. If it were possible to include in the statistics all these cases as well as those which are concealed because intentionally provoked, the frequency with which pregnancy is interrupted during the early months would be found somewhat greater than is usually supposed.

If we omit the miscarriages which occur within the first few weeks of pregnancy, and which consequently often escape detection, the majority of cases fall within the second and third months. After the fourth month has passed, the probability of such an accident, though not excluded, is greatly diminished. Some statistics recently published by Taussig make this clear. In a series of several hundred cases of miscarriage, one hundred and fifty-seven instances occurred in the second month, two hundred and twenty-two in the third month, seventy-three in the fourth month, thirty-seven in the fifth month, and five in the sixth month. This order of frequency might be anticipated from the anatomical conditions which prevail during the early months of pregnancy, since the attachment of the embryo to the mother is at first relatively insecure, but gradually grows firmer, and becomes as secure as it ever will be by about the fifth month.

It is noteworthy that miscarriage occurs much less commonly in the first than in subsequent pregnancies. Indeed, a somewhat greater liability to the accident with each succeeding pregnancy goes far toward explaining the greater frequency of miscarriage among women who have passed the thirty-fifth year than among those who are younger.

CAUSES AND PREVENTION.--We have seen that the proportion of pregnancies which end in miscarriage is quite formidable. But this should not be true, as the accident is frequently preventable, and many of these accidents could be avoided by the cooperation of patients. As self-denial and personal inconvenience are often essential, it is only fair to explain their value. Furthermore, the, patient who appreciates the reason for certain directions the physician gives becomes responsible to herself, and is much more likely to carry them out than is one who is cautioned without receiving a satisfactory explanation. At best, however, the advice which the physician is able to offer will be imperfect, for it must not be imagined that everything is known concerning the causation and prevention of miscarriage. While our knowledge is so imperfect we must be content to make the most of what we possess. It must be added that no suggestion such as can be given here will enable anyone to dispense with her own medical adviser. On the contrary, if there is reason to fear miscarriage, the prospective mother should be encouraged to seek his counsel as early as possible. Aside from the hygienic measures which she may learn to carry out for herself, various drugs are often of great value in preventing miscarriage. Since these are not applicable to all cases, they should be employed only upon medical advice.

Very early miscarriages may be explained by the loose attachment of the ovum during the first six weeks of pregnancy. This tiny, living sphere, it will be recalled, reaches the womb a few days after conception, and adheres to the uterine mucous membrane. At first, however, its roots are short and delicate, and not so capable of anchoring the ovum as they become later. It is only toward the end of the eighteenth week that the union between the womb and its contents becomes firm.

From what we have learned in Chapter II regarding the anatomical conditions in the early days of pregnancy it is obvious that we need not be greatly surprised at the frequency of miscarriage. On the other hand, it must not be forgotten that there are many natural safeguards against accident: to mention only one, the uterus is ingeniously swung in the abdominal cavity so as to afford a large measure of protection against mechanical shock. Usually, the provisions nature has made are sufficient to resist forces from without which tend to dislodge the ovum. Now and then it happens that the most irrational acts will not interrupt pregnancy; indeed, they often seem particularly inert when practised intentionally.

Fear of loosening the ovum from its uterine attachment prompts experienced women to caution prospective mothers against any kind of sudden or violent effort. Their advice, however, is often needlessly alarming; a great many traditional precautions lack a reasonable basis. Thus, no harm can possibly result from sleeping with the arms above the head; nor from "over-reaching," as when hanging a picture, though a fall under such circumstances might be dangerous.

Patients who have been warned by one experience should always be on their guard if they would avoid repeated miscarriages; others need only lead a sensible, hygienic life, a matter we have already discussed in the chapters dealing with the care of the body and the way to live. For the sake of emphasis, I may here repeat that no prospective mother should become fatigued from any cause; sweeping, moving heavy furniture, lifting heavy articles, and running a sewing machine are not to be attempted. But household duties which do not require strong muscular effort are better assumed than not.

Amusements which may cause jolting, or expose one to the danger of falling, involve some risk of miscarriage. Short rides in a carriage or an automobile over smooth roads are free from objection. Railway- travel and sea-voyages are not advisable in the early months; after the eighteenth week they may be undertaken with a greater degree of safety, provided comfortable accommodations are assured, and the patient has never had a miscarriage.

A few physicians, even at present, attribute the interruption of pregnancy to strong emotions, including intense joy or sorrow, anger, fright, or even jealousy. Without denying altogether the possibility of such an influence, we may be sure that its importance is greatly exaggerated. It is not unusual to see patients who are able to recall a mental shock of some kind shortly before the miscarriage occurred; nevertheless, in such cases diligent search will usually reveal a physical cause for the accident.

Another popular fallacy relates to the effect of drugs upon pregnancy. The use of castor oil and other strong purgatives do not interrupt it. Should the administration of any cathartic be followed by miscarriage, some fault inherent preexisted in the pregnancy, and no amount of precaution would have enabled the patient to reach full term successfully. Quinin in tonic doses may be taken with impunity, and even larger quantities are being constantly used for the cure of malaria without doing the pregnancy any harm. Many other drugs are reputed to have great efficacy in causing the expulsion of the product of conception; unfortunately, they are too well known to require enumeration. They are usually unreliable, and are absolutely inefficient in doses small enough not to endanger the mother's life, provided the pregnancy is a healthy one.

Instances in which miscarriage is attributed to the use of some drug are quite common, and we cannot dismiss them without a word of explanation. Such cases generally fall into one of two classes. Often a drug is given credit for efficiency where conception has been erroneously suspected. Shortly after the menstrual date passes, some medicine is resorted to, and the subsequent phenomenon, regarded as the interruption of pregnancy, is really no more than normal menstruation. In another group of cases miscarriage does actually occur, although the medicine employed plays only a minor role in its production. In such instances the irritation which the drug occasions is the last link in a chain of events leading up to the miscarriage, but the main factor lies in some fundamental imperfection in the pregnancy. Physicians recognize a variety of these imperfections, and know that they may be located in the womb, in the embryo, or in the tissues which unite the one with the other. As an intimate knowledge of pathology is often necessary to recognize the underlying, and therefore the actual, cause of the miscarriage, it is not at all surprising that patients frequently err in their interpretations of such accidents, and emphasize unimportant matters.

It would lead us too far afield to attempt to discuss every cause of miscarriage. Nevertheless, there are some very important ones, not yet mentioned, which should be understood by the laity, as appreciation of their significance may avert trouble. In some instances, on the other hand, the accident is unavoidable; to know this should afford the patient a large measure of comfort.

Irregularities in the position of the womb are often responsible for miscarriage. Such a condition may exist in women who have not borne children, but it is far more likely to occur as a result of childbirth. After delivery, the enlarged womb becomes the seat of intricate changes, the purpose of which is the restoration of the organ to the condition which existed before conception. It dwindles in size, and gradually drops to its accustomed location within the pelvic cavity. Six weeks are usually required for these changes.

At the time of birth it is impossible to predict whether the womb will finally resume a satisfactory position. Accordingly, an examination two to four weeks later is essential. In four out of five patients the organ will be found in its proper location, but, even though it is not, suitable measures adopted at once will generally serve to replace and hold it in good position. On the other hand, if the malposition is not recognized until months or years later, simple procedures will prove inefficient, and a surgical operation will become necessary. Were there no other reason for a careful examination at the end of the lying-in period, it would be amply justified by the information which it gives relative to the position of the uterus.

Although there can be no doubt that the routine correction of uterine displacements shortly after labor would go far toward restricting the occurrence of subsequent miscarriage, it would be incorrect to leave the impression that miscarriage will always occur if the uterus is out of its normal position. Not infrequently the changes wrought by pregnancy will cause the uterus to right itself spontaneously.

Another important cause of miscarriage consists in abnormalities in the lining of the uterus. Through inherent defect or acquired disease this tissue may become unsuited for anchoring or nourishing an ovum. In either event, a surgical procedure, known as curettage, affords the most likely means of restoring it to a healthful state. The operation removes the old lining; and a new one quickly develops, which is often more capable of fulfilling the purpose for which it is intended.

An appreciable number of miscarriages depend upon conditions over which medical skill has no control. Under such circumstances, though the accident may be regretted, there is no room for remorse or censure. Often the embryo should bear the blame; if its development is imperfect or if it dies, miscarriage usually occurs very promptly.

We are familiar also with a few maternal conditions which seriously affect the embryo, often seriously enough to cause its expulsion, alive or dead. In this respect, certain constitutional disorders are preeminent. Bright's disease and diabetes are prejudicial to the development of the embryo; women suffering from either of them must be watched with great care. Occasionally, such pregnancies come to a premature end in spite of every precaution. Various infectious diseases, as typhoid fever and pneumonia, also are fatal to the embryo if the causative bacteria pass into it. Fortunately this rarely happens, since the placenta generally affords an effectual barrier to their entrance into the embryo. Organic diseases of the mother's heart also may bring about miscarriage. A patient thus affected should place herself under the supervision of a physician as soon as conception is suspected.

Now and then physicians are completely at a loss to explain cases of miscarriage. Our ignorance is unfortunate, particularly when repeated miscarriages have occurred and their causation cannot be detected.

HABITUAL MISCARRIAGE.--Experience teaches that women who have had one miscarriage must be more careful than other prospective mothers if they would escape a repetition of the accident. Persons who know themselves to be subject to miscarriage should regard no precaution as too burdensome. Not only should they avoid motoring, driving, railroad journeys, sea voyages, and every kind of strenuous exertion, they must accept every opportunity to be quiet and rest. Often such hygienic care yields sufficient protection; but occasionally medicine is also necessary.

A number of causes are at hand to explain habitual miscarriage, but, in fairness, it must be acknowledged that physicians are not able to interpret all cases. With one class of patients the muscle fibers of the womb are peculiarly irritable, whereas in another its lining proves incapable of firmly anchoring the ovum. Moreover, derangements of organs which do not belong to the reproductive group may be responsible for the habit.

It is a curious fact that the accident is most likely to occur when menstruation would be expected were the individual not pregnant. Obviously, extraordinary precaution is advisable at such times, and if the patient would avoid even the slightest risk, she should not leave her bed. The same purpose will not be served by sitting quietly in a chair, nor by reclining on a couch; complete relaxation and composure are secured only when one lies flat on the back, loosely attired in sleeping garments. I have known several persons with a tendency toward miscarriage who overcame it in this way. Recently one of them who had been delivered prematurely on two former occasions, and who was anxious for a successful issue to her third pregnancy, was willing to remain in bed practically the whole period of gestation. She had her reward; a well-developed infant was born at full term, and has continued to thrive.

Prolonged rest in bed, some will say, is debilitating. While that may be true to a degree, untoward effects can always be avoided by systematic massage of the extremities. The abdomen should not be subjected to such manipulations, for they will occasionally provoke painful contractions of the uterus and defeat the purpose of staying in bed.

Patients who are not disposed to undergo a long period of enforced rest, no matter what profit may be promised, should at least consent to keep in bed during that period of pregnancy at which a previous miscarriage took place. We know that the event is particularly apt to recur at such a time. Specifically, it is important to remain in bed one week before and one week after the date in question.

When pregnancies follow one another in rapid succession, the liability to miscarriage is notably increased. A natural interval between births has been provided, an interval which depends upon the mother nursing her child. Ideally, menstruation, and with it the ripening of the ova (egg-cells), does not occur while the breasts are active; but when the infant does not suckle, the ovaries regularly resume their function in a very short time. Since the circumstances attending miscarriage always deprive the mother of the opportunity of nursing, another pregnancy may quickly ensue unless these facts are appreciated.

Those who anticipate the possibility of a premature interruption of pregnancy should realize that the marital relation is inadvisable after conception has taken place. For others, who have no reason to expect irregularity in the course of pregnancy, such a precaution is unnecessary. None the less, women who marry late in life or who first conceive toward the time of the menopause will do well to follow the same rule. The risk of accident may be very slight, but conservative persons will not assume it when the likelihood of subsequent conception is doubtful.

Not infrequently the fundamental reason for habitual miscarriage lies in some anatomical abnormality which a surgical operation alone can correct. As the necessity for interference can be determined only after a careful examination, recommendations of wide application are not possible. Nothing short of painstaking study of each case will afford a basis for advice and action.

SYMPTOMS.--Very definite warning usually precedes a miscarriage, but the threatening symptoms vary greatly in severity and duration. If appropriate measures are taken promptly, these symptoms may disappear with no harmful result Everyone concedes that bleeding and pain are the chief indications of impending miscarriage, although an occasional patient, profiting by former experience, may find other signs prophetic in her own case.

Mature women, accustomed to the regular monthly function of their sex, are prone to treat with indifference a slight discharge of blood occurring during pregnancy. Indeed, it is widely believed that menstruation frequently continues after conception. In point of fact, however, it is very unusual in early pregnancy, and becomes entirely impossible after the fourth month. Accordingly, whenever vaginal bleeding is noticed, some other explanation should be sought; and the patient who would adopt the wisest plan should assume that she is threatened with miscarriage. There are other possibilities, but these are for her doctor to consider.

It is true that small hemorrhages are not necessarily followed by miscarriage. One may even experience slight loss of blood repeatedly, and yet give birth to a healthy child at the natural end of pregnancy. None the less, bleeding, however moderate, should always excite suspicion, as we know it usually denotes the breaking to some degree of the connection between mother and child. The extent of the separation usually determines the degree of the hemorrhage, which in turn indicates the seriousness of the accident. The fate of the fetus will depend upon the area of placenta, which has been incapacitated. Flooding, however, always imperils the fetus, and generally warrants the inference that so much of the placenta has been separated as to render further development impossible. On the other hand, so long as the hemorrhage does not exceed the customary flow at the monthly periods, the life of the child is rarely endangered; while a chocolate-colored discharge, and even the loss of small clots, may continue indefinitely without doing serious harm. Under such circumstances, however, the patient should communicate with her medical adviser, and should save for his inspection whatever may be expelled.

Pain, the other conspicuous symptom of threatened miscarriage, has not a uniform significance. Since it frequently occurs during the course of pregnancy in association with a number of conditions, it is not a reliable sign of danger. Moreover, the susceptibility to pain varies; thus, of two patients in the same stage of threatened miscarriage one may suffer intensely, while the other remains comparatively comfortable.

Typically, the onset of miscarriage is attended by discomfort in the small of the back, which may be continuous, but more often is intermittent. If preventive measures are instituted at the outset, there is hope of relieving the discomfort and averting the miscarriage; but if the warning goes unheeded, the pain will gradually shift to the lower part of the abdomen and become more severe. It often happens that the cramp-like abdominal pain of threatened miscarriage is confused with that associated with intestinal indigestion. A simple test will sometimes decide the question. If due to the latter cause, the discomfort will usually yield to a teaspoonful of paregoric, whereas it will be without effect if miscarriage is imminent. Exceptions to this rule are not uncommon, yet a better one cannot be given; as a physician, even after considering the technical evidence, may find it impossible to decide at once whether or not miscarriage is threatened.

No confidence can be placed in many so-called signs of miscarriage, though implicitly trusted by the laity. Lassitude, depression of spirits, and general bodily ill-feeling may forecast the interruption of pregnancy; but more frequently they have no such significance. The same estimate holds true of other symptoms, including diarrhea and a persistent inclination to empty the bladder. Nor does fever always lead to the termination of pregnancy. A moderate rise of temperature is without significance; but high fever, persisting for several days, may result in the death of the fetus and subsequent miscarriage. Nevertheless, prolonged febrile affections, such as typhoid fever, frequently leave pregnancy unharmed.

So long as the symptoms are confined to slight bleeding and mild attacks of pain, physicians regard miscarriage merely as threatened. If the bleeding increases, the outlook becomes less favorable, and, as I have said, miscarriage is inevitable when it amounts to flooding. Likewise, rupture of the sack containing the fetus, with escape of the amniotic fluid, indicates that the culmination of events will not long be delayed.

The most favorable outcome is when the entire contents of the womb are spontaneously expelled, which unfortunately does not always occur. There is, to be sure, rarely any difficulty in the natural birth of the fetus, for its meager development prevents serious complications. The separation and extrusion of the placenta, on the contrary, are apt to be imperfect when pregnancy ends in the early months, and medical attention is necessary to determine whether the uterus has been emptied completely. This is particularly important, because the retention of placental tissue affords opportunity for several unpleasant complications; and neglect in this regard accounts in part for the belief that miscarriage is certain to leave women irreparably broken in health.

AFTER-EFFECTS.--No one will deny that invalidism follows the untimely interruption of pregnancy more often than the birth of children at full term. This is not due, as is sometimes said, to the fact that a miscarriage differs from a normal birth in that it is unnatural, for other reasons are apparent. One of them, the retention of placental tissue, has just been mentioned, but serious consequences resulting from it are almost inexcusable, for, although the placenta may separate less readily and be cast off less thoroughly after miscarriage, modern medical skill can successfully cope with such conditions. Another fruitful source of unfortunate after-effects is the imprudence of the patient. Women should remain in bed fully as long after a miscarriage as after the birth of a mature infant; if they would consent to do so, many ill-effects would be averted. But physicians frequently encounter strong opposition to precautionary measures such as this. Many patients argue, illogically, that less precaution is necessary since pregnancy failed to attain its natural conclusion, and infer that the earlier that it ends the more quickly one may leave the bed. In point of fact, even greater precaution is required than if all had gone normally. Still a third cause for ill- health may be found in physical ailments which antedated the miscarriage but were not recognized until after its occurrence.

Invalidism which follows pregnancy and which may be fairly regarded as chargeable to it depends, in most instances, upon an infection acquired at the time of delivery. Infection occurs more frequently when pregnancy ends during the early months, because in this category is included the great majority of criminal abortions, which are usually induced without regard for surgical cleanliness. Fatal complications, or serious consequences which narrowly escape a fatal ending, are common among women who attempt to rid themselves of an unwelcome pregnancy. As they are ignorant of aseptic precautions, their manipulations must necessarily contaminate the site of operation; for this reason and others as well women who attempt to perform an abortion upon themselves imperil their lives. The danger is scarcely less when abortion is induced unlawfully by incompetent operators; for lack of skill, the need of secrecy, and the desire of haste all interfere with necessary aseptic technique. Everyone knows that sad accidents befall those who submit to such operations; but it is not generally recognized that these cases are largely responsible for the ill-repute borne by miscarriage in general. On the other hand, properly supervised miscarriages are attended by no greater danger and probably less than delivery at full term.

CRIMINAL ABORTION.--The destruction of a pregnancy, except when its continuance threatens the life of the patient, is forbidden by law. The important ethical and religious aspects of the act which the law thus stigmatizes as criminal we may properly neglect. Although various religions present a diversity of teaching relative to its moral nature, all agree in regarding it as sinful. Equally important, however, is the fact that no matter what opinion anyone may hold as to the morality of the act he is bound to obey the law. This is apparently not clearly understood by the laity, for many persons think that a physician may terminate pregnancy whenever he is so inclined. If the liability to criminal prosecution which a physician would assume should he comply with a request for the means of destroying pregnancy were clearly realized, patients would not beseech him to incur the risk of heavy find and long imprisonment merely to gratify their own convenience or to save them from disgrace.

The Common Law, an inheritance from England, enriched with authoritative decisions by our own courts, is the groundwork of the law in all the States, and its principles are binding in the absence of express statutes. At Common Law, abortion is punishable as homicide when the woman dies or when the operation results fatally to the infant after it has been born alive. If performed for the purpose of killing the child, the crime is _murder_; in the absence of such intent, it is manslaughter. _The woman who commits an abortion upon herself is likewise guilty of the crime._

The great majority of those who desire the interruption of pregnancy feel they have not assumed an illegal position so long as they avoid instrumental procedures. That is not correct, for even at Common Law it is a misdemeanor to bring about the death of an unborn child by the use of drugs or by any other means.

At Common Law there was a difference of opinion as to whether all induced abortions were illegal. Many courts formerly held that quickening was a necessary prerequisite; but under the modern statutes, practically without exception, the law disregards the period of pregnancy at which the abortion is provoked. Since the time of conception determines the beginning of embryonic development, to prove that the act was committed before fetal movements were perceived is no longer a valid defense. This has been emphatically stated by Judge Coulter, of Pennsylvania, who said: "_It is not the murder of a living child which constitutes the offense, but the destruction of gestation by wicked means and against nature. The moment the womb is instinct with embryonic life and gestation has begun, the crime may be perpetrated._"

Each commonwealth has enacted its own statutes for the regulation of abortion. In many states, simply to seek the means for destroying pregnancy is a criminal act. Thus, Indiana, perhaps the most progressive of the States in reconstructing its criminal code to accord with modern sociological teaching, has enacted a law which I quote from Burn's Indiana Statutes, Revision of 1908, Vol. I, page 1029. "Every woman who shall solicit of any person any medicine, drug or substance, or thing whatever and shall take the same, or shall submit to any operation or other means whatever with intent thereby to procure a miscarriage, except when done by a physician for the purpose of saving the life of the mother or child, shall, on conviction, be fined not less than ten dollars, and be imprisoned in the county jail not less than thirty days nor more than one year." To include the woman as a party to the crime is a signal mark of progress toward bringing abortion under effective legal control. Heretofore, the perpetrator alone has been responsible, and in most States he remains so, while the woman is regarded as a victim. Clearly, that is unjust, for criminal abortions are rarely, if ever, performed without application by the subject of the operation. According to most of the statutes no distinction is made between the attempt at abortion and its accomplishment. Irrespective of the outcome, those who supply drugs or employ instruments purposing the destruction of pregnancy are guilty of the offense.

An extensive analysis of the various State laws is unnecessary; the mention of a few statutes, selected from different sections of the country, will suffice to indicate the character of prevalent legislation. Massachusetts imprisons those found guilty of abortion for a period of three years or less, and permits a fine of one thousand dollars. In Pennsylvania the same prison sentence is imposed, though the fine may not exceed five hundred dollars. Three years is the minimum imprisonment in Virginia, and a maximum of ten years is allowed. Colorado's law duplicates that of Massachusetts. California imposes no fine, and prescribes a sentence of from two to five years in the State prison. All the statutes make the offense much graver when the woman dies as a result of the practice. Under these circumstances, the crime never takes lower rank than manslaughter; and generally it is murder.

Evidently we possess sufficiently stringent laws regarding criminal abortion; yet, as everyone knows, they do not prevent perpetration of the crime. On good authority, we are informed that eighty thousand unlawful abortions are performed annually in New York, in spite of a possible penalty of four years in the State prison. This is due in part to difficulty in securing evidence and failure to prosecute when evidence could be gathered, but more particularly to the fact that the general public does not appreciate the gravity of the offense. The same feeling is illustrated in the advertising of abortifacients. Newspapers and magazines unhesitatingly carry, under the guise of remedies to regulate the health of women, notices of drugs and equipment intended to destroy pregnancy. This is expressly forbidden by many statutes. [Footnote: Thus, the Maryland law provides that "any person who shall knowingly advertise, print, publish, distribute or circulate any pamphlet, printed paper, book, newspaper notice, advertisement or reference containing words or language or conveying any notice, hint, or reference to any person or to the name of any person, real or fictitious, from whom, or to any place, house, shop, or office, where any poison, drug, mixture, preparation, medicine, or noxious thing or any instrument or means whatever; or from whom advice, direction, information or knowledge may be obtained for the purpose of causing the miscarriage or abortion of any woman pregnant with child, at any period of pregnancy, shall be punished by imprisonment in the penitentiary for not less than three years, by a fine of not less than five hundred dollars, nor more than one thousand dollars, or by both, in the discretion of the court."]

The knowledge that prohibitory laws exist is sufficient to deter reputable physicians from illegal practice; whereas known laxity in the enforcement of the law continually tempts unscrupulous persons to provoke abortion. Among the poorer classes the procedure is undertaken by ignorant women, while persons in more comfortable circumstances avail themselves of the services of medical men who are usually incompetent and value money above professional honor. The net result is an unpardonable death-rate and a large proportion of invalids. Aside from the legal aspect of the act, the element of personal danger would seem a warning to be heeded by women who contemplate becoming a party to this crime.

THERAPEUTIC ABORTION.--If a woman is suffering from tuberculosis or some organic affection, pregnancy may add a serious strain upon the already crippled machinery of her body. Occasionally gestation itself may cause changes which threaten life. In either event the duty of the physician is plain. The law is acquainted with such emergencies, and explicitly permits the termination of pregnancy when undertaken to relieve or cure such conditions. When performed to restore health the operation is called therapeutic abortion.

The Maryland law, for example, grants the right to induce abortion whenever two or more physicians see the patient and agree that "no other method will secure the safety of the mother." Similar rules are prescribed by the statutes of other States, but none concedes the right of abortion as a means of keeping the woman from suicide.

Since therapeutic abortions are legal, they may be done openly; hence the operation is performed in appropriate surroundings and with every refinement of surgical technique. These fortunate conditions materially alter the outlook; serious consequences of the operation itself need not be feared. Competent surgeons, employing modern methods, may perform hundreds of abortions without the loss of a single patient. Moreover, pregnancy may be terminated safely and expeditiously at any time; the lay view which regards abortion as more serious after the second month than before it is a relic of days gone by.

PREMATURE DELIVERY.--In the introduction to this chapter we noted that the infant becomes viable after the twenty-eighth week, which marks in a practical sense, the transition of the fetus from an immature to a premature stage of development. In point of frequency, premature delivery ranks far below either abortion or miscarriage.

Unlawful interference with pregnancy generally proceeds from a desire to avoid offspring, and lacks incentive after the infant becomes capable of living independently. Criminal operations, therefore, are not a conspicuous cause of premature delivery. Occasionally physicians resort to artificial means to end gestation during the later months in order that organic complications may be relieved; but most premature births occur spontaneously. Sometimes they are due to ill-health, while in other instances no evidence of disease is found in either mother or child. Careful study of the individual patient, however, is generally helpful toward the prevention of repeated premature delivery.

The course of premature labor closely resembles delivery at full term. But it is shorter because the infant is small; and the subsequent loss of blood is not so great. The recovery of the mother is never retarded by the fact of earlier delivery, though the conditions which caused it may prevent rapid convalescence.

The outlook for the infant depends upon a great many factors. Most important among them is the perfection of its development, which may be estimated most satisfactorily from its weight and length. Occasionally children have been reared when they weighed as little as three pounds, but hope that they will survive should not be entertained unless they weigh four pounds or more. This is attained about eight weeks before maturity, and corresponds to a length of forty centimeters (16 inches), measured from the crown of the head to the heel. Premature children perish, most frequently, either from incomplete development of their heat-regulating apparatus, which predisposes them to pneumonia, or from imperfections in the digestive functions, which increase the liability to malnutrition. To overcome the first danger, incubators have been devised and have become familiar to everyone through public exhibitions. A basket or box supplied with hot-water bottles answers the same purpose, and has the advantage of better ventilation. The second danger can be overcome only by proper feeding. Breast-milk provides the most reliable nourishment for premature infants. If the mother cannot supply it, a wet-nurse should be procured, and, if the infant has not the strength to suckle, the milk should be drawn from the breast and fed with a medicine-dropper or a spoon.

In addition to providing proper food and maintaining an even body-temperature, care must also be taken to protect these infants from various harmful influences such as too much handling, strong light, and loud noises. Although every precaution be observed, frequently all counts for nothing; but if the child does thrive, there is no reason for worry about its ultimate development. When a premature infant lives, the same chances for adult health await it as it would have had if born in its due time.

CHAPTER IX

THE PREPARATIONS FOR CONFINEMENT

Engaging the Nurse--Desirable Qualities in the Nurse--Preliminary Visits of the Nurse--The Necessary Supplies for Confinement--The Baby's Outfit--Sterilization--The Choice and Arrangement of a Room-- The Bed--The Preliminary Visit of the Doctor--When to Call the Doctor--Personal Preparations--The Care of Obstetrical Patients at the Hospital.

Prospective mothers are anxious to learn how they shall prepare for the approaching confinement. They desire their preparations to be thorough, reliable, and in accord with the most approved methods of treatment, for they realize that preparations along these lines will not only prevent haste and confusion at the time of birth, but will also promote a satisfactory convalescence. Apparently trivial details often safeguard confinement against serious accident. Indeed, measures which aim at the prevention of illness form the chief asset of modern obstetrics, and of these none takes higher rank than the maintenance of strict cleanliness during and after childbirth. This fact fortunately is widely appreciated at present, and not a few women inquire voluntarily the means of observing the proper precautions. It is true, of course, that even today many women are delivered in filthy rooms and upon dirty beds, and that in spite of such surroundings some of them make a good recovery. Yet grave complications develop much more frequently among those who have not paid attention to the preparations for confinement.

The surgical dressings and other supplies do not require attention in the early months of pregnancy. A number of articles, invaluable when delivery occurs at full term, are useless if the fetus is immature and cannot live, and therefore it is unnecessary to provide them until two or three months before the confinement is expected. In the event of a miscarriage what is needed can be procured upon very short notice. But, on the other hand, delivery subsequent to the twenty- eighth week may require all the equipment useful at full term so that everything should be in readiness by that time.

ENGAGING THE NURSE.--As soon as the existence of pregnancy is clearly recognized the patient should select the doctor and the nurse who will attend her. Prompt selection of a nurse will assure the widest choice, for proficient nurses are in demand and book engagements far in advance of the date they will be needed. Furthermore, it is a relief to the patient to have her attendants selected. The possibility of premature delivery never interferes with engaging the nurse very early in pregnancy, for that accident releases both patient and nurse from their contract.

Nurses demand that the date be specified upon which an engagement shall begin, as, unless their calendar is definitely arranged, they are unable to earn a livelihood. This leads to a question which is difficult to answer, for the precise day of delivery is uncertain; consequently to fix the beginning of the engagement may prove a troublesome matter. On the one hand, there is risk of having to pay the nurse for a time before her services are actually needed; on the other, a false economy may result in the absence of the chosen nurse at the critical moment. In finding a way out of this dilemma a patient must be guided by her means and the location of her home. Those who can afford it will not hesitate to employ a nurse from one to two weeks in advance of the expected date of confinement; and for those who live where nurses cannot be procured quickly, a similar course is recommended. But persons of only moderate resources, living in a city where, in an emergency, a substitute can be gotten from the local "Nurses' Directory," will find it convenient to engage the nurse from the calculated date. The substitute will remain with the patient until the arrival of the nurse originally engaged.

Occasionally, it may happen that a patient will prefer to keep the substitute. Such a course, however, would be unjust to the nurse who was first selected, unless she could immediately secure other work. She has reserved a definite period of her time for the patient, and probably has declined work which seemed likely to conflict with the engagement already made. She is fairly entitled, therefore, to assume charge of the case, and the patient who refuses to make the change is obligated to pay her according to the terms of the agreement.

How long will a nurse be needed after the child is born? The answer to this question may be altered by so many circumstances that a hard and fast rule cannot be given. Before the advent of "Trained Nurses," obstetrical patients were cared for by "Monthly Nurses," so called because they remained one month with their patients. It is, likewise, customary to keep the trained nurse four weeks after the birth; but whenever possible it would be well to retain her six weeks, since this period elapses before the mother has entirely regained her normal physical condition. Those who can afford to keep a trained nurse six months or a year are exceptional, but very fortunate.

Someone may feel that the suggestions I have made are not suitable to her case. Very likely they may not be; to cover all the possibilities could scarcely be expected, for every case has its problems and peculiarities. After consultation with her physician each patient will decide what is particularly advisable for her. Nevertheless, I would emphasize the importance of securing a competent nurse and retaining her for at least four weeks. Even with those who must guard their expense account the truest economy will lie in such a course. Whenever lack of resources seems likely to prevent this arrangement, the patient who is looking to her best interests should enter a hospital where excellent care can be provided at a cost within her means.

DESIRABLE QUALITIES IN THE NURSE.--It is rarely advisable to select as nurse a member of the family or an intimate friend. Some of the motives governing such a course--sentiment, mutual devotion, and the desire to be humored-- are inconsistent with the best kind of nursing. If the nurse knows the patient intimately, undue anxiety may interfere with her judgment; thoroughness in routine duties may be hindered by mistaken consideration for the patient; and in an emergency sympathy rather than reason may guide her. A successful nurse must satisfy at least two requirements; she must be capable professionally and also personally agreeable to her patient. Some regard advanced years as essential to the first of these qualifications, but this does not necessarily hold good.

The personal qualities generally welcome in a nurse are neatness, thoughtfulness, a sympathetic nature, an even disposition, and a cheerful view of life. Since a short interview is insufficient for taking the measure of a nurse, patients usually rely upon the opinion of someone else in selecting her. The judgment of her former patients is frequently prejudiced in one direction or the other, and such an estimate must always be accepted with caution. Much the most trustworthy method is to allow the physician to select her. He will know nurses who possess the requisite qualities, and certainly he is most competent to judge their professional attainments. If the choice of a nurse be left to the doctor, the two are sure to work harmoniously, and the patient will benefit by their cooperation. Otherwise she may suffer because of their dissensions, for, if the doctor is accustomed to one procedure and the nurse to another, misunderstandings may occur, although both methods yield equally good results. Whenever he does not select her, she should be asked to confer with him long before the case is due. Obviously, a physician cannot be held responsible for a nurse's ability unless he is acquainted with her training and methods of work.

In an effort to economize, many are inclined to employ "half-trained" or "practical nurses." When the confinement is not the first and there is no reason to anticipate any irregularity during labor or thereafter, I can see no vital objection to such an arrangement. It is of the first importance, however, to be assured that the "practical nurse" is neat and appreciates the necessity of keeping everything about the patient scrupulously clean. But competent nurses who charge less than the customary fee will be hard to find. The recommendations which these women receive are apt to be even more misleading than in the case of trained nurses, because more is expected of the latter. My experience has taught me that patients form particularly unreliable opinions of practical nurses, and I have frequently witnessed incompetence in such women which was overlooked by the patient.

A low-priced nurse is seldom a cheap one, as her shortcomings may be reflected in the health of the mother or the infant long after she has left the case. Especially when the baby is the first, the mother will depend upon the nurse for instruction which should be both sound and thorough. The principles taught her will be put into practice and utilized for many months, playing a vital part in the training of the infant. It becomes essential, therefore, to secure a nurse who will give the baby a good start, and instruct the mother along right lines. Perhaps this is less needful if the mother has learned her lesson from previous experiences. But even then a good nurse relieves her of responsibility and materially assists her to a quick and lasting convalescence. In the end the most proficient nurses are the least expensive.

THE PRELIMINARY VISITS OF THE NURSE.--Many of the precautions which safeguard a confinement should be considered by the patient and the nurse together. The character and quantity of the supplies, the choice of a room for delivery and subsequent convalescence, the proper clothing for the infant--all these are problems which may be solved most satisfactorily in the light of the nurse's experience and the resources at hand. Two visits are usually sufficient to arrange these details. An interview early in pregnancy, soon after the nurse has been selected, provides an opportunity to lay plans and especially to review the list of articles needed at delivery. Such articles as are already in the house may be checked off; the others may be procured at leisure. Eight to ten weeks before the expected date of the confinement the nurse should pay a second visit and should inspect the supplies to see that they are complete. Certain articles which I shall indicate must be sterilized. As this procedure is more reliable when carried out by an experienced person it will be convenient to have all the dressings finished by the time of the nurse's second visit, in order that she may sterilize them.

The question may arise as to whether the nurse shall come to the patient upon the date for which she has been engaged or shall wait until summoned. From the physician's standpoint it is often more acceptable to have the nurse in the house a few days before the confinement, though some patients strongly object to this. Provided the nurse may be got quickly at any time of day or night, there can be no objection to leaving the decision to the patient herself.

THE NECESSARY SUPPLIES FOR CONFINEMENT.--As to just what a confinement outfit should contain physicians differ to some extent; but this disagreement pertains rather to luxuries than essentials. In the lists here suggested nothing essential has been omitted, although economy, as far as is consistent with good judgment, has been kept in mind. Any article not included in my list which the doctor or nurse in attendance recommends may be noted in the space for memoranda.

Some patients prefer to take no part in preparing the supplies for confinement. Indeed, the demand for a ready-made confinement outfit has become large enough to lead several firms to put them upon the market. These outfits differ in completeness and vary in price from a few dollars up to fifty. The majority of patients, however, still attend to such details themselves, and will find a list of the needful supplies convenient.

Make-up and Sterilize: 7 Dozen Sanitary Pads. 2 Sanitary Belts. 2 Delivery Pads. 5 Dozen Gauze Sponges. 2 Dozen Gauze Squares. 4 Dozen Cotton Pledgets. 2 Sheets. Bobbin for tying the Cord. A Pair of Obstetrical Leggins. A Dozen and a Half Towels (Diapers).

Obtain from the Druggist: 100 Bichlorid of Mercury Tablets. 100 grams Chloroform. 4 ounces Powdered Boric Acid. 4 ounces Tincture Green Soap. 1 pint Grain Alcohol. A small jar of White Vaselin. A cake of Castile Soap. A two-ounce Medicine Glass. A Medicine Dropper. A bent glass Drinking Tube.

The following articles should be in the house, ready for use.

An ample supply of Towels, Sheets, and Gowns.

A new Hand-Brush; the cheap variety with wooden back and stiff bristles is preferable.

Two slop Jars or enamel Buckets with Covers.

A two-quart Fountain Syringe; an old one may be substituted provided it has been thoroughly boiled.

Three Basins and a one-quart Pitcher of agate or enamel-ware.

A Douche-Pan; the "perfection Bed-Pan" is preferable.

Two pieces of Rubber-Sheeting are required, one large enough to cover the mattress of a single bed (2 x 1-1/2 yds.), the other smaller (1 x 3/4 yd.). Should this be too expensive, the best substitute is white table oil-cloth.

The nurse will explain how the various surgical dressings are made, but, as the patient may forget some of the directions, all the details will be given here. At least three to four pounds of absorbent cotton will be used in the dressings. To make the pads entirely of absorbent cotton is very expensive. The cheaper cotton- batting is therefore employed to give them body, and they are faced only upon one side with the absorbent material. Furthermore, the rolls of absorbent cotton, as purchased, may be separated into three or four layers, one of which is thick enough for the facing. About six rolls of the batting should be purchased.

Surgical gauze, which tradespeople sometimes call dairy-cloth, is the most suitable material for covering the pads. Bleached cheese cloth will answer the same purpose, but it is more expensive and rather heavy. Approximately thirty-five yards of the gauze, which comes in a thirty-six-inch width, will be needed. When the supplies are finished, they are wrapped in separate bundles and sterilized. Old muslin or some of the diapers are generally used for covers.

The sanitary pads, also called vulval or perineal pads, absorb the discharge which always occurs after delivery. They are made of absorbent cotton and cotton-batting covered with gauze; a convenient size is ten inches long and three to four inches wide. Their thickness is approximately an inch, one-third of which is composed of absorbent cotton.

The sanitary belt is used to hold these pads in place. Very satisfactory ones are made of two strips of unbleached muslin, three inches wide. The first of these must be long enough to reach around the waist; the second, which passes over the pad, is somewhat shorter and has two parallel slits in one end; through which the waist-band passes at the back; the three free ends are pinned together in front.

The delivery pads are made of the same materials as the sanitary pads; preferably a yard square and four inches thick. A rather heavy top-layer of absorbent cotton must be used in them, and they should be quilted or tacked at several points to prevent slipping. A rubber pad is ill adapted for use during delivery. Some absorbent material made into proper shape proves much more satisfactory since it can be thoroughly sterilized and can be thrown away after it has been used.

I am told that cotton-waste is a good substitute for absorbent cotton in the delivery pads. It is inexpensive, and will be rendered capable of absorbing fluids after it has been boiled in washing soda and dried in the sun. Each delivery pad should be separately wrapped and sterilized.

Gauze sponges will be needed by the doctor; about five dozen should be prepared. The gauze is cut in eighteen-inch squares. Opposite edges are folded toward one another, about two inches being lapped each time; this finally yields a seven or eight-ply strip, which is wrapped into appropriate shape about two fingers. The ravelled ends are then tucked into the roll. It is most satisfactory to divide the sponges and sterilize them in two bundles.

Small pieces of gauze about two inches square will also be needed in caring for the baby's eyes and mouth. Several dozen should be cut, and they may all be sterilized together.

Cotton pledgets are simply bits of absorbent cotton the size of a hen's egg, the rough edges of which have been twisted together. A small pillow-case full of them ought to be made up and sterilized.

Obstetrical leggins are preferably made of canton flannel; they are cut to fit loosely and should reach the hip. If they are prepared so as to extend to the waist at the sides, they may be held in place by a waistband, and in this way will prevent unnecessary exposure without interfering with the doctor. They should be sterilized.

Towels, if used at all, should be without fringe. It is economical not to employ them, but to use diapers in their place. Three packages, each containing six diapers, should be sterilized.

Sterilized sheets are often useful at the delivery; more than two are never needed. They should be wrapped separately for the sterilization.

Sterilized bobbin is generally used for tying the cord. Several pieces are cut in nine-inch lengths and sterilized in a single package.

A dressing for the cord will be required, but there is no necessity for preparing a special one. It is generally satisfactory to wrap the cord in one of the sterile gauze sponges which has been previously soaked in alcohol.

Several methods of drying up the cord give equally good results, and it is usually a good plan to allow the nurse to dress it as she wishes, since the employment of a method with which she is familiar will more likely insure a satisfactory result in her hands. A dressing popular with many nurses is prepared as follows: In a piece of muslin four inches square cut a small circular opening; double the linen and dust boric acid between the folds. If this method is preferred, several of the dressings should be prepared and sterilized together.

THE BABY'S OUTFIT.--Preparations for the infant may be thorough without being elaborate. Instinctively, the prospective mother leans toward extravagance in fitting out her baby's wardrobe, and easily slips into the error of providing too much. Time and energy are frequently devoted to an extensive wardrobe which the infant quickly outgrows; in consequence many articles must be made over before they are used. Even with modest resources a prospective mother can acquire everything the baby really needs.

A very sensible plan, in my judgment, is to prepare what will be wanted during the first two months; subsequently, articles may be made or bought as they are needed. Accordingly, the quantity of wearing apparel and the nursery supplies I have suggested pertain only to the early weeks of infant life. Although no essential has been omitted, the outline is plain and economical.

At present, outfitters supply a variety of ready-made, garments for the infant and conveniences for the nursery; in many of them notable ingenuity is displayed which aims at the child's comfort or the saving of labor to the mother. Catalogs of these articles, which are often expensive, are furnished by dealers.

In preparing clothing for the new-born, several principles must be kept in mind. The first is that the garments must be warm without being unduly heavy; and another that they should be roomy, permitting perfect freedom of motion. A third no less important principle is simplicity. Adornment of the clothing gratifies the mother, but does not serve a single useful purpose. The lists which follow include all that is necessary for the young infant; they will also serve as a basis for elaboration if a more lavish outfit is desired.

Necessary Clothing. 4 Abdominal Flannel Bands. 3 Undershirts. 4 flannel Skirts. 4 Night Gowns. 12 White Slips. 3 Knit Bands. 4 Dozen Diapers. Cloak and Cap.

Nursery Equipment. An old Blanket. Assorted Safety Pins. Soft Damask Towels. Wash Cloths. Hot-Water Bag with Canton Flannel Covers. Talcum

Powder. Olive Oil. Bassinet.

Additional Articles; Convenient but Not Essential. Rubber Bathtub. Rubber Bath-Apron. Flannel Apron. Bath Thermometer. Bath Hamper. Quilted Mattress Covering. Baby Scales. Screen. Low Chair without Arms. Drying Frames.

STERILIZATION.--Now and again, those who follow very rigid rules to avoid infection during childbirth are criticized for their pains. The general public has not yet grasped the true relation of bacteria to this condition; a relation which, indeed, first became clear to medical men within comparatively recent years. The development of our knowledge of the nature of infection forms one of the most entertaining chapters in obstetrics, and provides a simple way of showing the genuine need of preventive measures. Several observant physicians had previously suspected the character of "child-bed fever" (as infection of the mother was once called), but convincing proof of its contagious nature was not forthcoming until the middle of the nineteenth century, when signal facts were pointed out by three men, each working independently, though all came to similar conclusions. The evidence they gathered should have left no one doubtful that the disease is contagious, and largely preventable. On the contrary, bitter opposition was encountered for the time, and only within the last two decades has their teaching found wide practical application.

In 1843 Oliver Wendell Holmes published the paper on "The Contagiousness of Puerperal Fever," which is now preserved in his volume of "Medical Essays." Physicians were startled to be frankly told the responsibility they assumed if they neglected the truth taught by epidemics of this disease. "The dark obituary calendar" which marked the progress of these epidemics clearly indicated that "the disease is so far contagious as to be frequently carried from patient to patient by physicians and nurses." A violent controversy followed this arraignment, and, consequently, the preventive measures which Holmes so convincingly urged were not adopted as promptly as they should have been. The full justice of his conclusions has since been universally admitted, and medical men now find it difficult to understand how anyone could have taken issue with the sentiment which he expressed. "For my part," Holmes said, "I had rather rescue one mother from being poisoned by her attendant than claim to have saved forty out of fifty patients to whom I had carried the disease."

But the most important early observations upon child-bed fever were made in 1847 by a young Hungarian, Semmelweiss, while he was an assistant in the large Lying-in Hospital in Vienna. In thoroughness, power of conviction, and practical value his work was masterful. It is no exaggeration to regard his observations as the rock upon which antiseptic surgery, the glory of the nineteenth century, was built.

Semmelweiss had been seeking an explanation of the dreadful scourge, and his mind was ready for the reception of the truth when it was revealed through the death of one of his colleagues. This physician injured his finger accidentally in performing an autopsy upon a patient who had died from child-bed fever. And the condition disclosed by examination of his body after death was identical with that found in cases of child-bed fever. Here then was the clew; the disease was contagious. Semmelweiss was ignorant of Holmes' views; what had happened before his eyes suggested to him that the disease was due to a poison which could be conveyed from one person to another. Moreover, his interest and his power of insight led to further comparison. Clearly, the open wound on the physician's finger had been the portal through which the poison entered; but where was there a similar portal in obstetrical patients? The answer was plain. The birth-canal at the time of delivery is always an open wound. There the poison entered, and child-bed fever was a wound infection!

Several years later Tarnier, who was to become an eminent obstetrician, but was then a student in Paris, chose the diseases of the lying-in period as the subject for his graduating thesis. He was unacquainted with the work either of Holmes or of Semmelweiss, and approached the problem from still another standpoint, drawing attention to the much higher deathrate among women delivered amid unsanitary surroundings. Tarnier also considered that the disease was a form of poisoning, that it was contagious, and that measures should be instituted to protect patients against it.

Of these pioneers, by far the greatest credit is due Semmelweiss, who devoted his life to the problem, although his opinions continually met with scepticism and even ridicule. More convincing proof than he could furnish was demanded before his contemporaries would believe that child-bed fever was due to lack of precaution. Fortunately the evidence was soon produced. In 1880, Pasteur obtained bacteria from the organs which had been infected, and was able to grow the bacteria in his laboratory; thus the ultimate cause of the disease became firmly established. With the harmful agents in their hands, Pasteur and his followers were enabled to study their characteristics and to recommend means of destroying them.

Much as we must regret that the warnings of Holmes and of Tarnier passed unheeded; lamentable as may be the blindness of the generation of Semmelweiss to the truths revealed by his research, it is not surprising that such radical teaching met with a hostile reception. As we measure time in retrospect from the vantage ground of to-day, the three to four decades required for full acceptance of their revolutionary doctrines seem a brief span. Antiseptic methods would not have prevailed so quickly as they did, had not the same epoch which gave us a Pasteur also given a surgeon with a receptive mind, ready to seize and apply the discoveries of the French genius. This was the great service of Joseph Lister. Impressed with Pasteur's studies on fermentation, Lister saw an analogy between this process and the putrefaction of wounds, a condition which he was eager to prevent. He had reason to believe that carbolic acid would check decomposition, and he employed a weak solution of it in the treatment of wounds; later he devised a "carbolic spray," by means of which when his operations were performed the atmosphere round about might be sterilized.

It is but a short step from antiseptic operations to our own era of aseptic surgery, and that a step in the direction of simplicity. Now we know that the sterilization of the air is rarely necessary and have dispensed with Lister's elaborate apparatus. Furthermore, and of far greater moment, experience has taught that the destruction of bacteria before they have opportunity to come in contact with the wound is more effective than efforts to kill them as they approach or after they have invaded the tissues. Initial freedom from bacteria is the ideal of asepsis; to secure it, the modern surgeon is ever watchful of the cleanliness of his hands, his instruments, his dressings, and of the site of operation or whatever may come near it.

The importance of the changes wrought by the adoption of aseptic methods requires no emphasis, for the marvels of modern surgery are even more impressive to laymen than to the medical profession. Everybody now understands that strict cleanliness is indispensable to the success of a surgical operation. But the general public has not fully awakened to the same profound necessity in connection with childbirth, although it was child-bed fever that called forth the observations and experiments upon which modern surgical technique rests.

Although most obstetrical patients appreciate the fact that there is an advantage in sterilized dressings and sanitary surroundings, few realize the risk they run without them. One must know the mournful history of the past to be adequately impressed with that danger, for we no longer see the epidemics of childbed fever which formerly swept over communities, sacrificing ten of every hundred women as they became mothers. Precaution is no less necessary on that account; the scourge would be rampant again if the reins were loosened.

Most instances of puerperal infection are, it is true, referable to lack of care. Nevertheless, the complication develops now and then where all precautions have been conscientiously observed. Under such conditions the infection will in all likelihood be a mild one, and a tedious convalescence usually proves its most disagreeable feature. Such stringent preventive measures as are now practiced in many hospitals have reduced the frequency of infections to the point where only one fatal case, or even less, occurs in a thousand deliveries. These rare cases remind us that vigilance must never be relaxed, and that patients who are confined at home require just as much care as those in hospitals, where conditions are the best to prevent infection and the complications, which follow.

The first essential toward the avoidance of infection in obstetrical cases is clean dressings. Naturally, these should be clean to the sight, but it is in invisible dirt that serious danger lurks; bacteria are the causative agents of this disease. Experiments have taught the bacteriologist that disease-producing organisms are killed in half an hour when subjected to a high atmospheric pressure and the temperature of steam. Special apparatus has been constructed for carrying out the procedure. It is unnecessary for our purposes, however, since the essential conditions may be secured, though with less convenience, in any kitchen. If a prospective mother finds it awkward to do the sterilizing at home, and her nurse is unable to take charge of the matter, she may arrange with a local hospital or the nearest nurses' directory to sterilize her dressings. Yet a very little ingenuity suffices to do the work at home with perfect satisfaction. Installments of the smaller bundles may be sterilized in a galvanized bucket. To do this place an inverted bowl, with a depth of three to four inches, at the bottom, and pour in water until the bowl is almost covered. A breakfast plate rests on the bowl, and upon this the dressings are stacked; a second larger plate which fits the top of the bucket is utilized as a lid to close in the sterilizing chamber. This will not accommodate the larger packages; a more satisfactory method for all of them is to use a wash-boiler in which has been swung a muslin hammock.

To arrange the latter form of home sterilizer, cut an oblong piece of unbleached muslin large enough to sink far down into the boiler and run a drawing-string of stout cord about the edge. Cover the bottom of the boiler with several inches of water; tie the hammock in place, passing the cord beneath the handles of the boiler to hold the muslin securely. Pack in the dressings, which have been wrapped in appropriate bundles; put the lid in place, thus closing the sterilizing chamber, and leave the dressings exposed to the steam for at least half an hour. After the operation has been completed, the bundles are taken out of the boiler and allowed to dry in the air. They must not be opened until the occasion for which the supplies were prepared arrives; awaiting this event, they are laid away in a convenient closet or drawer.

A word of caution may be added concerning a method of sterilization employed at home more frequently, perhaps, than any other. According to this procedure, the supplies are wrapped in paper, thrust into a hot oven, and left there until the paper is scorched. From the standpoint of economy as well as of thoroughness, this method is likely to prove unsatisfactory. Frequently, the dressings themselves are scorched; I have known patients to ruin several installments of their supplies in this way. Moreover, dry heat is not so trustworthy as steam for sterilizing purposes.

Judicious management means the preparation of the supplies necessary for confinement before turning to the selection of the infant's outfit. Ordinarily, both these tasks should be finished by the end of the eighth month, and final arrangements for the approaching delivery will then claim attention. If the patient expects to remain at home, she must decide which is the best room to occupy; she will wonder how it ought to be equipped, and she will be anxious to learn what personal preparations are advisable at the beginning of labor.

Intelligent answers to these questions are important. A patient should request the physician to criticize her plans when he pays the preliminary visit four to five weeks prior to the expected date of confinement. If she has acted unwisely in any respect, he will point it out, and may suggest changes which will enable her to employ to the best advantage the resources at hand.

THE CHOICE AND ARRANGEMENT OF A ROOM.--An old-fashioned custom, which relegated obstetrical patients to the most secluded part of the house, with little regard for comfort and still less for hygiene, has now few, if any, adherents. There is an advantage, to be sure, in having a quiet room; but this qualification may be secured in a room well located with regard to other essentials. Selection of a suitable room is not a trivial point. In most cases, since patients ordinarily remain for convalescence in the same room in which the infant is born, the chamber must serve a two-fold purpose. A number of requirements, therefore, must be met, and they must all be kept in mind when the room is chosen.

We have seen that the act of birth, natural as it is, may have a very unnatural sequel if precautions against infection are treated lightly. It is proper, therefore, that the delivery-room should be as clean as care can make it. Such radical measures as may be employed in sterilizing the dressings are here out of the question; if possible, they would be absurd. Infection usually develops because harmful bacteria come in contact with the patient. For that reason, an infection is more likely to be communicated by the dressings than by articles about the room, which only become a source of danger when the dirt upon them is transferred by an attendant.

An acceptable delivery-room may be arranged in any home; it is by no means necessary to duplicate the equipment of a modern hospital. To choose a room convenient to the bathroom will be found advantageous not only at the time of birth but throughout the lying-in period. The furnishing should be simple and scrupulously clean; indeed, it is improbable that one of these good points can be secured without the other. Furthermore, the preparation of the room should be completed well in advance of the date of confinement.

A large collection of furniture interferes with the nursing, and also increases the difficulty of keeping the room free of dust. It is sound advice, therefore, to remove everything which will not serve some good purpose during the delivery. Should any article be wanted later, it can be brought back to its accustomed place. The furniture may be conveniently limited to a bed, a bureau, a washstand, a table, and several chairs, one of them a large, comfortable rocker, which will prove invaluable during the early part of labor.

To approach perfect conditions, bric-a-brac, needless hangings, and everything that might collect dust should be temporarily removed. A profusion of pictures does not accord with the best sanitation of a room devoted to the treatment of obstetrical patients; those which are to be left upon the wall ought to be taken down and wiped carefully with a damp cloth. Other desirable preparations would be instinctively undertaken by the modern housekeeper, and it may seem presumption to mention that the room itself ought to be subjected to most thorough cleaning. It is well to leave the floor bare or merely covered with freshly cleaned rugs. Carpeting is difficult to protect against soiling and is not sanitary. If left down, the carpet should be covered with some suitable material, firmly stretched and tacked in place.

We know that the air in most households does not contain disease-producing bacteria; but the presence of any contagious disease materially alters the situation, and may imperil the convalescence of an obstetrical patient. Preferably, one should never select a room in which there has lately been sickness, and under no circumstances may such a room be used until carefully fumigated. The more conspicuous diseases which for at least several months absolutely disqualify an apartment for obstetrical purposes are diphtheria, pneumonia, pleurisy, erysipelas, scarlet fever, typhoid fever, tuberculosis of all varieties, and every sort of discharging sore.

When possible, two adjoining rooms should be given over to the mother and the infant; if this is impracticable, the single room should be large, easily ventilated, well lighted, and heated in such a way as to permit a change of temperature without difficulty. All these features help to make convalescence comfortable and free from petty annoyances. A room which has a southern or eastern exposure proves grateful for those who must remain indoors; frequently, this will be beyond reach, but a room getting the sun's rays directly during part of the day will always be available, and the selection should be made with that requirement in mind. At the time of birth and for the first few days which follow, a patient may not appreciate this feature; ultimately she will understand the need of sunlight better than the need for the more technical, and therefore the more impressive, preparations.

THE BED.--Now that housekeepers recognize how easily such furniture can be kept clean, few homes are without a brass or an iron bedstead; they are equally sanitary. Undoubtedly, this kind of bedstead fulfills the needs of an obstetrical patient much better than any other; and, if at hand, it should be used. The single bedstead is the most acceptable, and the mattress ought to be at least twenty inches above the floor. A low, wide bed interferes with proper management of the delivery and later handicaps the nurse in taking care of the patient. Wooden blocks may be used to raise a bed which otherwise would be too low. It is well worth while to provide them if one desires good nursing, for no attendant can do her best when she must continuously bend over a very low bed.

The location of the bed at the time of delivery is not an unimportant matter; it must always be placed so that the brightest possible light will shine over the foot. Since birth often occurs at night, one should make certain that the artificial lighting of the room is good, and place the bed most advantageously in reference to it; at the same time the necessity of a good light from the windows, when delivery occurs during the day, should not be forgotten. The head of the bed may be placed against the wall, but both sides must remain freely accessible not only at the time of delivery but also throughout the lying-in period.

A smooth, firm mattress, made in one piece, should be provided. One which has been used several years and possibly worn in a hollow will require renovation to be made comfortable. A feather bed should not be used under any circumstances. The mattress must be protected; and protection is best secured by means of a large piece of rubber sheeting. The regulation household sheet covering the rubber should be tucked well under the mattress at the ends and sides; in that way the rubber sheeting will be held firmly. Since the part of the bed where the hips rest will be most exposed to soiling, the protection of this area is usually reinforced by a "draw sheet." To arrange this, a cotton sheet is doubled so as to make a strip about one yard wide and two yards long; the smaller piece of rubber sheeting is laid between the folds. The draw sheet will reach from the middle of the back to the knees; its ends should be tucked under the sides of the mattress, to which it is fastened by means of large safety pins. After delivery, the draw sheet may be removed without disturbing the mother, who will thus be assured a clean, dry, and comfortable bed.

The bed-clothes covering the patient during labor will vary with the season of the year, but should always be light; in summer a single sheet will suffice, and in winter a blanket will likely be needed. For sanitary reasons, a freshly laundered sheet should also be placed outside the blanket until the delivery has been completed; later, it may be replaced with a light spread. Two pillows will be needed, and it is very convenient to have one of hair, the other of feathers. While there is no necessity for sterilizing the bed-clothes, it is advisable to use linen which has been recently laundered and kept well protected from dust. Among the poor, infection from soiled bed- linen is not uncommon.

THE PRELIMINARY VISIT OF THE DOCTOR.--No teaching of medical science has been given greater prominence of late than the principle of prevention. In obstetrics it finds a particularly wide field of application, and its practice is responsible for removing many of the former terrors of childbirth. We have just learned that preventive measures effectually reduce the frequency of puerperal infection, and in an earlier chapter we saw the value of routine examination of the urine as a means of anticipating other complications. Moreover, the benefit of promptly reporting to the physician anything that does not seem to be as it should has been urged constantly, for in this way is afforded the earliest opportunity to treat complications. Similarly a visit from the doctor about four weeks before the expected date of confinement is indispensable to skillful management of the delivery; neglect of this precaution is sometimes responsible for bad results.

At this visit the physician not only becomes familiar with the general health of his patient, but he also notes certain facts which will have a direct bearing upon the course of labor. By means of a few simple measurements he may accurately determine the character of the pelvis, the bony structure through which the fetus passes. When they are compared with what we know as the normal measurements, a very good idea is gained as to whether the birth-canal will present any obstacle to the passage of the child; and, if it will, there is opportunity to deliberate what treatment may be necessary. Since another factor in the problem, namely, the size of the child, cannot be accurately predicted, occasionally the physician may hesitate to express as definite an opinion as the patient may wish. Nevertheless, though it may be impossible to learn every detail, the available information well repays the time and trouble expended. In nine out of ten cases nothing whatever is found out of the way; the result is an assurance which always justifies the examination.

During this examination the position of the child is also ascertained. By means of a series of painless manipulations through the abdominal wall of the mother, the head, the body, and the extremities of the child may be mapped out, and the conclusions verified by locating the fetal heart-sounds. In this regard, also, the physician usually finds normal conditions. The most favorable presentation, that in which the head is the part to be born first, occurs in ninety-seven of every hundred cases. When less favorable conditions are recognized, they may frequently be corrected at once; but should that prove impossible, with foreknowledge of the presentation, the physician will be more competent to conduct the delivery.

With a clear understanding of the character and value of the information gathered at the preliminary examination, patients are not likely to refuse it. If they do, the risks should be fully explained to them. Some physicians decline to assume the responsibility of a patient who will not permit these observations. Such a decision is rarely necessary, for in my experience the patient's consent has never been difficult to obtain. Many women now regard the visit as part of the routine attention, and inquire when it will be made.

The appropriate time for this examination, as I have indicated, is approximately one month prior to the calculated date of confinement. Before this period, we have no assurance that the presentation which is found will continue until the time of birth. The fetus frequently alters its position as long as it is not large enough to fill out the cavity of the womb, consequently it is only during the last month of pregnancy that the final presentation can be determined. But to defer the examination after the period I have specified is unsafe since we lack an exact method of fixing the day of confinement, and too long a delay might render a preliminary examination impossible.

Aside from its relation to the observations just outlined, the preliminary visit provides an opportunity for the physician to criticize the preparations which have been made, and for the patient to inquire about the personal preparation advisable at the beginning of labor. She will also learn the signs which indicate that labor has begun and will be told what to do when they appear. Although physicians may not agree in all these directions, there can be no difference of opinion relative to the essential points. At least, the rules given here will serve to bring the patient and the doctor to a definite understanding as to the course he desires her to follow.

WHEN TO CALL THE DOCTOR.--During the last two or three weeks of pregnancy not a few patients are more comfortable than they have been for several months. About this time the womb usually drops somewhat and relieves the pressure which has interfered with breathing. These changes, however, do not promote comfort in every direction; more freedom for the organs of the chest means compression of the structures below the womb; consequently, the inclination to empty the bladder and for the bowels to move becomes more frequent. Patients complain also of cramps in the legs and experience difficulty on walking. This order of events enables some women to recognize the approach of delivery. Of course there is other evidence when labor actually begins. Its onset may be indicated in one of three ways, namely, by periodic pains, by a gush of water from the vagina, or by a discharge of blood as though the patient were taken unwell. Each of these unmistakable signs is a sufficient reason for notifying the doctor.

At the onset of labor, dragging pains are usually felt at the back, but sometimes in the lower part of the abdomen. The rhythm with which they come and go identifies them more certainly than any other feature, though this indication is not entirely reliable, for intestinal colic also causes rhythmical pain. At first the uterine contractions which occasion the discomfort are weak and appear at long intervals. Gradually they become stronger and closer together. When the interval between them has been shortened to half an hour or less their significance is fairly certain, provided the abdomen becomes tense and hard with each pain, remaining comparatively soft between them.

When contractions begin during the day or early evening, the physician will be glad to have immediate notification in order that he may arrange his appointments and thus be free to attend the patient when she needs his services. On the other hand, if they begin between 11 P.M. and 7 A.M. the nurse, who will always be summoned with the very first warning, should be allowed to decide when the doctor is to be called. Unless other instructions have been given, she will usually wait until the interval between the contractions is five to ten minutes.

Usually the symptoms make it clear that labor has begun, but occasionally the greatest difficulty will be experienced in deciding whether the discomfort has not some other origin. Uncertainty may prevail not only because of the similar effects of colic, but also from the fact that uterine contractions do not always have the same value. Preliminary pains may appear several days, or even weeks, before the actual onset of labor. Now and then the "false" pains cease, and after a period of comfort efficient contractions are established. There is never difficulty in recognizing the latter; doubt always relates to the preliminary pains, which may subside or may pass into the efficient type. We lack a method of foretelling which turn they will take; developments may be calmly awaited, with the assurance that ample warning will precede the birth.

A slight mucous discharge from the vagina is frequently seen toward the end of pregnancy and may be disregarded, but a gush of watery fluid always means that the sac which contains the fetus has ruptured. Uterine contractions generally follow within a few hours, though in a few instances they will not appear for a number of days. Under any circumstances the event ought to be promptly reported to the doctor. Similarly, he should be notified whenever bleeding from the vagina occurs, since it is important to have him determine its significance.

Anyone who supposes that patients are more likely to be infected when delivery occurs so quickly that there is not time for the doctor to arrive overlooks the leading factor in the production of this complication. Unless harmful bacteria are introduced into the birth- canal and lodge there, infection is impossible. Bacteria never enter of their own accord; they are usually carried into the vagina by means of an examining finger or some other foreign body. Accordingly, with the exception of those instances in which local inflammation already exists, there is no reason to fear infection when delivery proceeds so rapidly that internal examinations are not required.

PERSONAL PREPARATIONS.--Ordinarily, if the nurse is not already in the house, she will arrive in time to assist the patient in making the final arrangements for delivery. Should the nurse be delayed, the patient herself may make certain preparations to insure personal cleanliness, another very important factor in the prevention of infection.

The presence of hair and the folding of the skin about the outlet to the birth-canal render the disinfection of this area somewhat difficult. It is advisable, therefore, to clip the hair as short as possible and, while bathing the whole body, to scrub the region in question with especial thoroughness. Before the bath an enema of soap-suds should be taken to clear the rectum of material which otherwise might be expelled during the birth and contaminate the field of delivery. The bath-towels and the gown which are used should have been freshly laundered.

Other especial preparation of the delivery-field will be made later by the nurse. But whenever labor progresses so rapidly that neither the nurse nor the doctor arrives before the child is born, such preparations as I have indicated will be sufficient, for more minute precautions are unnecessary unless an internal examination must be made.

THE CARE OF OBSTETRICAL PATIENTS AT THE HOSPITAL.--The majority of obstetrical patients are attended at home, and there is no reason why this should not be. Generally it is unfair to urge a woman to go to a hospital if she has already passed through a normal confinement and there is no reason to anticipate trouble in the approaching one; on the other hand, if any complication whatever is anticipated, the patient should certainly enter a hospital. Furthermore, it frequently proves advantageous to do so where the pregnancy is the first, though no complication is expected and none develops. The average labor with the first child lasts somewhat longer than with subsequent ones, and in consequence there is greater opportunity for the patient's family or friends to interfere with the management of the case, which never benefits a patient, and is sometimes a serious handicap. Then again, the cramped apartments, so common in these days, are poorly adapted to the treatment of sickness of any sort and should induce many obstetrical patients to choose the hospital. There are, besides, other features which favor this course, such as economy, convenience, and safety. From my own experience, which includes the care of patients both at home and at the hospital, I am convinced that, as a rule, the latter is much more satisfactory.

Most cities now have institutions which provide a room and all the essential care, exclusive of the doctor's services, at approximately the cost of a trained nurse at home; luxuries will naturally add to the expense in hospitals as quickly as elsewhere. If one considers the various items connected with attention at home, such as the maintenance of the nurse and of the patient, the cost of the equipment necessary for confinement, the additional household laundry, and the sundry other details, it is clear that hospital treatment becomes distinctly economical. Moreover, the uncertainty of the date of confinement may necessitate paying a nurse for a longer or shorter period before the birth. Expense at the hospital, on the contrary, usually begins when the patient enters; and if she lives in the city it is rarely advisable for her to leave home until the beginning of labor. Even aside from the matter of expense some women prefer the hospital, since in this way they avoid the technical preparations for the birth.

Much more vital, however, is the care patients receive in the hospital, for rigid adherence to surgical cleanliness is exemplified in the hospital as it can be nowhere else. Infections rarely develop there. Formerly these accidents were more common in the hospital than in the home, but conditions are now reversed and fatalities predominate among those delivered in private houses. The modern theory of asepsis has, to be sure, been widely accepted and is practiced so far as possible wherever obstetrical patients are attended, but only in the hospital can the underlying principles be applied with complete thoroughness and persistence. The hospital is constantly alert, whereas in private houses carelessness or ignorance, or both, often lead to lax technique. As a result, statistical evidence indicates that two to three infections occur among those delivered at home for one at the hospital.

In the event of an emergency during labor, the hospital affords another distinct advantage in its staff of trained attendants. Of course they may be brought to one's home, yet not without some delay and extra expense; whereas in the hospital their assistance is instantly available. In institutions charity patients are often delivered under more favorable auspices than are the wealthy at their homes. Convalescence likewise is favored at the hospital, since the rules which control the admission of visitors guard the mother from exhaustion and annoyance. Moreover, isolation such as can only be secured in a hospital is conducive to a well-trained baby.

Patients debating what course to follow often ask when they must leave home, what they should take with them, and how long they ought to remain at the hospital. The attending circumstances will alter the answers to these questions, but in a general way the following directions will serve as a guide.

Ordinarily, the patient may remain at home until the first warning of labor. Departure from this rule is justified if the patient becomes unduly anxious about reaching the hospital in time, especially when she lives some distance from the institution, or if there is any doubt of securing accommodations. In either event, she should go to the hospital at least one week before the confinement is expected. There is no danger in riding to the hospital after labor has begun; frequently, the ride exerts a helpful influence and shortens the labor.

Whatever is to be taken to the hospital should be packed in a bag several weeks before the predicted date of confinement and put in a convenient place so that one may be spared the trouble of gathering it at the last minute. Beside her usual toilet articles, the mother will require several gowns, a dressing-robe, and bedroom slippers. Clothing for the child will also be needed since most institutions stipulate that the infant use its own wearing apparel. If impracticable to transport the entire wardrobe when the mother enters the hospital, so much may be taken as will be needed during the first few days, and other articles may be brought as the need of them arises. The personal laundry of both mother and infant is usually done outside the institution.

Surgical dressings of every description are provided by the hospital. Those who intend to enter a hospital, therefore, may disregard the list of articles necessary for confinement. Similarly, the sterilization, the preparations of the room and of the bed, and personal preparations will be of interest only to the patient who intends to stay at home.

It is not always possible for the physician to say how long a patient should remain at the hospital; the rapidity of the mother's convalescence and the progress of the child, both important factors, cannot be accurately foretold. Frequently, it is a good plan to remain until the infant is four weeks old, but the majority of patients are dismissed at a somewhat earlier date. In no instance, however, should the mother be allowed to leave before the infant is two weeks old. Even when given the privilege of leaving so early she will always understand that competent assistance must be provided at home, for the mother should not resume her routine duties until six weeks after the birth.

CHAPTER X

THE BIRTH OF THE CHILD

The Cause of Labor--The Course of Labor--The Stage of Dilatation--The Stage of Expulsion--The Placental Stage--The Effect of Labor upon the Child--Meddling--Justifiable Intervention--Management of Birth without the Doctor--Methods of Reviving the Child.

The birth of a child is an act of nature, an act generally performed as satisfactorily as any other bodily function. Birth has, however, so deep a meaning for the mother, as well as for her family and her friends, and is, above all, so vital to the future of the race, that it has naturally become the subject of many impressive superstitions. Primitive peoples have invariably embodied in their religion their views of the origin of life and the phenomena of its inception. With these mysteries Greek and Roman mythology dealt extensively, as did also the myths of the Phoenicians, the Egyptians, the Chinese, and the people of ancient India. No race, indeed, has lacked its own interpretation of childbirth, and no phase of the process has failed to have attributed to it a supernatural significance. A number of these superstitions still distress women on the eve of motherhood. To correct exaggerations and to deny many utterly false impressions of childbirth there is no better way than to give a frank account of what does actually occur. I shall adhere to a purely physiological description of the event, for, although I appreciate fully the fact that its sociological and sentimental aspects are perhaps equally important, these are not, in my opinion, pertinent to a medical discussion.

In a scientific sense the act of birth may be described as a series of muscular contractions which widen the birth-canal and expel the contents of the pregnant womb. Since the process requires an expenditure of energy, it has come to be called labor. Intrinsically, labor does not differ from many other physiological acts. The heart drives blood into the arteries; the bladder empties itself; the intestine moves its contents and finally expels the undigested residue. All these acts strongly resemble that of birth; but they also differ from it, for the head of the fetus is a hard body which resists being molded to the shape of the passageway through which it enters the world. To this resistance the pain which accompanies delivery is largely due. And yet even in this respect the act of birth is not unique; certain circumstances lead to painful contractions of the muscle fibers in the intestine and less frequently of those in other organs.

It is natural to ask what purpose is served by the pain associated with labor; and a moment's reflection will make it clear that one reason for the discomfort is the warning which it gives of the approach of birth. If the mother were not thus cautioned, she might be delivered under very awkward circumstances, and even under such conditions that occasionally the infant would perish the instant it was born. All mammals suffer in giving birth to their young, though with quadrupeds the period of suffering is shorter, for the upright posture of man has changed the shape of the pelvis, rendering birth somewhat more difficult. Anyone who observes the lower animals preparing for delivery will be convinced that they also are responding to pain, the most compelling call of nature.

That the suffering is at all essential to the mother's love for her child I cannot believe. Under certain circumstances, as for example when the Cesarean operation is performed before the onset of labor, the delivery is painless; yet I have never known a mother less devoted to her child on that account. Biology throws no light upon the relation of the "curse of Eve" to present-day confinements.

THE CAUSE OF LABOR.--It is evident that, in a general way, the muscular contractions of the womb cause the birth of the child; but before we thoroughly understand the act, science must discover what stimulates the muscle to contract. Although careful research has thus far failed to disclose the source and character of the stimulus, it has taught many properties of the contractions themselves. Their force has been measured and found to increase as the end of labor is approached; the pressure they exert varies between nine and twenty- seven pounds. We also know that the patient can neither hasten nor delay the contractions voluntarily. Strong emotions are believed to accelerate them at times, and we find a very extraordinary illustration of this effect recorded in I Samuel, IV, 19, where we read: "Phineas' wife was with child, near to be delivered; and when she heard the tidings that the ark of God was taken, and that her father-in-law and her husband were dead, she bowed herself and travailed; for her pains came upon her." On the other hand, and much more familiarly, excitement checks the contractions after they have begun. Every obstetrician has heard patients say that with his arrival the pains died down. Yet such an influence is never permanent; the contractions soon reappear, and labor advances as though no interruption had occurred.

For the artificial induction of labor, the physician has at his disposal means that resemble the method sometimes employed by nature. Suitable appliances introduced into the womb provoke contractions, and labor proceeds step by step as if the stimulus were a normal one. Nature does not, however, ordinarily employ mechanical irritation to start the uterine contractions. The initial factor is more remote and, as I have said, is not yet well understood.

Since, as everyone admits, delivery occurs with conspicuous regularity about the end of the fortieth week of pregnancy, and pregnancy corresponds, therefore, to ten menstrual cycles, some have been led to believe that labor and menstruation have a common basis. The truth of this supposition, however, must be doubtful until we know the cause of menstruation. Yet it is a matter of common observation that the uterus becomes unusually irritable about the time when the tenth menstrual period would be due. Strong purgatives administered with other drugs on or after the calculated date frequently bring about delivery, whereas previous attempts of this kind prove unsuccessful. To account for this peculiar irritability of the uterus about the fortieth-week of pregnancy, microscopical changes in its tissues have been suggested but sought in vain. Nor will the distention of the organ explain it.

A great many theories have been offered to explain the causation of labor, but they have now only an historical interest. To-day we are just beginning to learn the correct methods of studying the problem. The experience of ages has firmly established the fact that the fetus is expelled when ready to enter the world, or as we say, when it has become mature. But how does the fetus assert its maturity? There is the kernel of the matter; that is the real problem, a problem for the solution of which, happily, we possess better facilities than have heretofore existed. One solution that has been suggested assumes that the fetus loses ultimately its power to assimilate the nourishment provided through the mother's blood. In consequence, it is argued, the material which previously enabled the fetus to grow now collects-- in the maternal circulation, stimulating the womb to contract.

A part of this explanation, namely, that the material which stimulates the muscle fibers, whatever it may be, is a chemical substance and that it circulates in the mother's blood, is almost certainly true. There are, however, very weighty reasons for believing that this substance has not the character of food. A more plausible supposition is that the fetus produces this material in the course of its natural living processes, and the substance would accordingly be a waste-product.

THE COURSE OF LABOR.--The current view that labor begins in the early evening and generally ends during the night is incorrect. This impression has grown out of the fact that the whole process frequently consumes twelve hours and must in such an event include some part of the night. Statistical evidence indicates that almost as many births occur at one hour of the twenty-four as another; to be precise, only five per cent. more children are born between 6 P.M. and 6 A.M. than between 6 A.M. and 6 P.M.

As already pointed out, labor commonly begins with transient discomfort in the lower part of the back. At first the uterine contractions are far apart; they last but a moment and cause only twinges of pain. Gradually, the preliminary contractions give place to others of more definite character, which appear at intervals of five to ten minutes. Estimates of the total length of labor will vary according as one counts from the first warning or from the advent of typical contractions which we hear called "pains of the right kind." These generally continue for about four hours, and this period represents the average length of time the physician remains constantly with his patient. Estimates which include the initial symptoms are longer, varying from ten to eighteen hours. Prolonged labors are rare; and extremely short labors are also infrequent, though now and again it will be only an hour or two from the very first pain until the child is born.

To predict absolutely the length of labor for any particular patient is impossible. The averages calculated from large groups of cases have no more than a broad scientific interest; when applied to any individual they are apt to be very misleading. Thus, from statistics we should expect the first labor to be longer than subsequent ones, but we are often surprised by an unusually rapid delivery.

To facilitate description, labor is divided into stages which are conveniently designated the first, the second, and the third. During the first stage the way is prepared for the expulsion of the child; at the end of the second stage the child is born; the third stage is occupied with the separation and the expulsion of the after-birth. The progress of labor may be ascertained from time to time by means of suitable examinations. Whereas formerly vaginal examination was the only method which served this purpose, we are now acquainted with several. For example much of the information necessary for the proper management of delivery may be gained from examination of the patient's abdomen; and this may be supplemented by observations too technical to consider here.

Occasionally I have heard doctors accused of negligence because they failed to make numerous vaginal examinations. Censure of this kind generally is unjust, for discretion in limiting the number of vaginal examinations provides against infection a guarantee which cannot be overestimated. In many cases, of course, they are still invaluable toward determining what treatment should be pursued, yet they are never employed to the extent once customary. Moreover, physicians have learned to take extraordinary precautions whenever vaginal examinations must be made.

Anyone who practices obstetrics in these days appreciates how careful he must be, especially of the cleanliness of his hands. Energetic scrubbing with soap and water and the free use of antiseptics, as physicians now employ both these measures, appear ridiculous to some women who have witnessed deliveries under a less stringent regime. They may be bold enough to express their disapproval. They may remind us that many women have been successfully delivered without such care. And in this they are correct; we know that nine of every ten mothers passed through childbirth uneventfully before modern precautions were dreamed of. Such precautions as are now taken, however, are necessary to secure the safety of the tenth patient. And it is because they are anxious that all their patients shall enjoy the greatest possible security that physicians dare not omit any precaution.

Disinfection of the physician's hands does not entirely exclude the danger of infection through vaginal examinations. Although he may have been most conscientious, there is some risk of carrying contaminating material into the birth-canal from the region about the opening of the vagina. Unless that region has been satisfactorily disinfected, sterilizing the dressings and cleansing the hands may become a waste of time. Sensible patients, therefore, will never object to the preparations which the nurse is instructed to make.

THE STAGE OF DILATATION.--For reasons which are sufficiently clear, the womb must remain closed while fetal development is in progress; but under normal conditions, when this development is complete, the mouth of the womb dilates and the infant is expelled. The infant never takes an active part in its birth, although physicians once thought it did and attributed tedious labors to stubbornness on its part. The error has been corrected in medical teaching, but many persons unacquainted with the facts cling to the idea that the infant forces its own way out of the womb.

At the end of pregnancy the mouth of the womb is small, too small, often, to admit an instrument as broad as a lead pencil. It is obvious, therefore, that very radical changes must be wrought before the infant can pass. The door, as it were, must be widely opened. This phenomenon, which we call dilatation of the womb, is brought about by involuntary contractions of the muscle fibers in its wall, every point of which they draw upward. Now, the top of the womb is directly opposite its mouth, consequently the contractions inevitably pull its lips wider and wider apart. Ordinarily another factor is concerned in this mechanism. To understand the whole process we must recall that a fluid surrounds the fetus, and that this fluid is contained within elastic membranes. The uterine contractions compress the fluid, drive the membranes, like a wedge, into the mouth of the womb and spread its lips apart. Thus, to the pulling effect just mentioned, a pushing force is added. After full dilatation has been accomplished and the membranes can serve no further purpose, they rupture; as the midwife puts it, "the bag of waters breaks." The quantity of fluid which escapes will vary. Occasionally, a huge gush will drench the patient's clothing; but more often what is lost at first amounts to only a few teaspoonfuls, though small quantities of fluid often dribble away with subsequent contractions.

Although not the rule, it is by no means unusual for the membrane to rupture at the onset of labor, or at least before the mouth of the womb is fully dilated. Exceptionally, rupture occurs a few days before labor begins; and still longer intervals, though extremely rare, have been recorded. Whenever the membranes rupture prematurely, the pushing force of the uterine contractions becomes less effective, though the pulling force is never impaired. Under these circumstances, which occasion what is called a "dry labor," delivery is apt to proceed slowly, yet that does not follow necessarily, for the part of the fetus which happens to lie over the mouth of the womb may act as efficiently as the unruptured membrane would.

During the first stage, the longest of the three, the patient is comfortable between the contractions and generally interests herself in some diverting occupation. The presence of the physician can be of no assistance then, and patients rarely demand it. Usually, they are satisfied to know he is ready to come when called. It is wrong to deceive patients with various recommendations from which they will vainly expect help during this stage; their welfare is best served when they are left alone. Generally the advice of well-meaning friends will be as harmless as it is futile, yet I must emphasize that during the first stage straining to expel the fetus is ill advised. Such effort will surely be ineffective then and may exhaust the patient; in that event it becomes harmful, for she will be fatigued when she most needs strength.

Since, during the first stage, the progress of delivery is not influenced by what the patient may choose to do, she may follow her own inclinations. The average patient will be restless and will keep on her feet most of the time; alternately she will walk or stand still as one or the other happens to make her more comfortable. As a contraction begins she often seeks support, leaning upon a chair or bending over the foot of the bed, and presses with her hands against the lower part of her back. Patients may sit down or lie down whenever they wish; if so inclined they may even go to sleep.

Most patients take no food during the whole course of labor, but, if nourishment is desired, there is no reason for abstaining from it. They may always drink water as freely as they like, and may also have milk, weak tea or coffee, or broth; but alcoholic beverages should never be taken without the specific consent of the physician. This same caution applies to strong coffee and tea. If desired, crackers or toast and rice or other cereals may be eaten in reasonable quantity. For fear of vomiting a patient will occasionally be told not to partake of any food. This advice is given, not because the symptom is alarming, but to save her needless annoyance. Indeed, vomiting frequently indicates that dilatation is well advanced, and, therefore, may generally be regarded as an encouraging sign. Ordinarily a persistent inclination to have the bowels move has the same significance. On the other hand, a constant desire to empty the bladder is more prominent at the onset of labor than later.

To know the moment which marks the transition from the first to the second stage of labor can be of no benefit to the patient; but for the medical attendant the greatest interest centers about this point. Casual observation sometimes enables the physician to recognize it, for characteristically at the close of the first stage the whole picture changes. In a typical case the membranes will rupture at this instant, expulsive efforts will begin, and, as we have just learned, there may be symptoms referable to pressure. Moreover, a blood-tinged discharge, spoken of as the "show," usually makes its appearance about the same time. Since slight bleeding frequently occurs at the beginning of labor, or a little later, this manifestation, like all others, may not be implicitly trusted to indicate the end of the first stage. Such uncertainty, however, is a matter of no great consequence, for in the absence of all these symptoms the physician may, if necessary, accurately determine the degree of dilatation by an internal examination.

THE STAGE OF EXPULSION.--The term delivery has been broadly applied to include the whole of labor. More strictly, its use should be limited to the second stage, for this period alone is concerned with the actual birth of the child. Although dilatation has been completed, the uterine contractions continue, devoting their force to emptying the womb. In this they now receive assistance from the voluntary contractions of the abdominal muscles.

The second stage is very much shorter than the first; for this reason and others, too, it proves much less trying. As the child is moved downward through the birth-canal, the mother usually appreciates for herself that she is making headway; whereas in the first stage she may know of progress only through what she is told. Moreover, it is possible in this stage for the physician, by means of inhalations of chloroform, to relieve her of the pain attending the expulsion of the child.

 Since the anesthetic properties of chloroform were discovered by an obstetrician who was searching for a drug with which to lessen the pain of childbirth, the facts connected with the discovery have a peculiar interest for mothers. Sir James Y. Simpson had always been anxious for some means to prevent the suffering endured during surgical operations "without interfering with the free and healthy play of the natural functions." He, therefore, welcomed the introduction of ether anesthesia from America; and in January, 1847, at the Edinburgh Medical School, administered ether to an obstetrical patient. This was the first instance in which an anesthetic was employed at the time of childbirth. Since ether, to his mind, had certain shortcomings, Simpson set about finding another anesthetic, and devoted all his spare time to testing the effect of numerous drugs upon himself. How he came to try chloroform has been vividly told by one of his neighbors. [Footnote: "Late one evening, it was the 4th of November, 1847, Dr. Simpson, with his two friends and assistants, Drs. Keith and Duncan, sat down to their somewhat hazardous work in Dr. Simpson's dining room. Having inhaled several substances, but without much effect, it occurred to Dr. Simpson to try a ponderous material which he had formerly set aside on a lumber- table, and which, on account of its great weight, he had hitherto regarded as of no likelihood whatever; that happened to be a small bottle of chloroform. It was searched for and recovered from beneath a heap of waste paper. And with each tumbler newly changed, the inhalers resumed their vocation. Immediately an unwonted hilarity seized the party--they became bright-eyed, very happy, and very loquacious--expatiating upon the delicious aroma of the new fluid. But suddenly there was talk of sounds being heard like those of a cotton mill, louder and louder; a moment more, and then all was quiet--and then a crash! On awakening, Dr. Simpson's first perception was mental--'This is far stronger and better than ether,' said he to himself. Hearing a noise, he turned round and saw Dr. Duncan beneath a chair, quite unconscious, and snoring in a most determined manner. More noise still and much motion. And then his eyes overtook Dr. Keith's feet and legs making valorous attempts to overturn the supper table. By and by Dr. Simpson having regained his seat, Dr. Duncan having finished his uncomfortable and unrefreshing slumber, Dr. Keith having come to an arrangement with the table and its contents, the sederunt was resumed. Each expressed himself delighted with this new agent, and its inhalation was repeated many times that night. Miss Petrie, a niece of Mrs. Simpson, gallantly took her place and turn at the table, and fell asleep, crying: 'I'm an angel! Oh, I'm an angel!'"--Quoted from "The Life of Sir James Young Simpson," by H. Laing Gordon; Masters of Medicine Series.]

The introduction of chloroform met with violent opposition, not upon medical grounds alone, but also for moral and religious reasons. "To check the sensation of pain in connection with the visitations of God," zealous theologians announced, "was to contravene the decrees of an all-wise Creator." Simpson reminded them "that the Creator, during the process of extracting the rib from Adam, must necessarily have adopted a somewhat similar artifice--for did not God throw Adam in a deep sleep?" Nevertheless, a number of years passed before the prejudice against artificial sleep was overcome. Chloroform only became popular after Queen Victoria consented to its use at the birth of her seventh child, Prince Leopold, in 1853.

There is still some difference of opinion regarding the routine employment of chloroform in obstetrical practice, though the weight of authority favors its use during the contractions at the end of the second stage, providing always that no preexisting organic derangement renders the drug dangerous. Under no circumstances, however, should chloroform be given in the first stage, and seldom at the beginning of the second. Prolonged administration will exert an injurious influence upon both mother and child; under these conditions it ultimately weakens the uterine contractions and delays the delivery. Such an effect must be avoided, since it would endanger the life of the child by asphyxiation as well as exhaust the mother. On the other hand, a few drops of chloroform inhaled with each pain toward the end of the second stage will dull sensibility, although consciousness remains unaffected. When the drug is thus administered, the uterine contractions are scarcely, if at all, altered, and the assistance which the patient is willing to give herself generally becomes more powerful. Should the anesthetic have the opposite effect, it must be withheld; but that is seldom necessary. As the head advances the anesthesia is deepened, and the mother sleeps soundly while the child is being born.

As long as dilatation is in progress, the patient may sit up or walk about; but with the advent of the second stage she should go to bed, for there she will be able to make the best use of the expulsive pains. The appropriate posture for delivery is still the subject of dispute, though modern views in no instance advocate the unnatural absurdities formerly supported by custom or superstition. Students of ethnology relate that among savage tribes almost every conceivable position was advocated for women in labor. Subsequently it became customary to have delivery take place in specially constructed chairs which are still used in semi-enlightened countries. With civilized nations at present women are always delivered in bed; yet national peculiarities still prevail. Some physicians favor what is known as the English position, in which the patient lies on her left side with her face inclined toward the chest, the trunk bent toward the knees, and the legs drawn up toward the abdomen.

The Britain revelleularly and completely. Nevertheless, so long as a mother is nursing her child she must be careful to keep the breasts in a healthful condition. They require support, yet must not be compressed. And they should be covered with clothing which will adequately protect them from sudden changes of temperature. This latter precaution, perhaps, requires more emphasis than formerly, on account of the present popularity of motoring; for the chill which one experiences when driving fast may have a very unpleasant effect upon a nursing mother unless her breasts are carefully protected. Occasionally fever and neuralgic pains in the breasts are caused by motoring, or by exposure to the air-current from an electric fan playing directly upon them. But even under these circumstances an abscess need not be feared unless the nipples are sore.

Human Milk.--Between the time of birth and the beginning of lactation there is always an interval during which the breasts secrete colostrum, just as they do throughout pregnancy. Although the nutritional value of this fluid is not great, it is doubtful if colostrum serves any other essential purpose than as nourishment. Possibly it also stimulates the intestines to expel the material which has collected within, them during fetal development, yet we know the bowels will move without a purgative; and often do so long before the infant is placed at the breast. Typically, the secretion of milk begins the third day after delivery; yet in perfectly normal patients it may appear as early as the second or as late as the fifth, and occasionally lactation does not begin until the baby is more than a week old.

As to what starts the secretion of milk we have only a vague idea; but we know that when the flow is once established its continuation depends primarily upon the sucking efforts of the infant. If nursing is discontinued the secretion dwindles and the breasts dry up. On the other hand, the strong, persistent stimulus of the infant's suckling gradually brings the secretion to a high degree of efficiency. Within the first two weeks, therefore, the daily secretion increases from a few ounces to a pint or more. Subsequently the output fluctuates between one and two quarts daily, according to the demands made upon the breasts; the secretion is larger, consequently, if there are twins. Astounding yields of milk have been recorded, as in the case of a wet-nurse in a German institution who nursed a number of infants and became capable of supplying three to four quarts daily.

That newborn infants thrive better on human milk than on any other nourishment is a conviction that must come home to every one who has had even a limited experience. It keeps the babies in health, serves to make them grow, and promotes the development of all their organs as nothing else will. Because there are present in this fluid all the elements necessary for nutrition, physiologists have called it a perfect food. Quantitatively its most important ingredient is water, which constitutes about 86 per cent. of its weight. It also contains about 7 per cent. of milk-sugar, 4 per cent. of butter fat, 2 per cent. of protein, and 0.2 per cent. of mineral matter.

The milk of all animals contains a relatively small quantity of mineral matter; judged from this standpoint, the mineral matter would seem of minor importance, but it is actually as vital as any other constituent. Without it the bones would hot harden properly; and other services which it performs are absolutely essential to life. As we should expect, human milk contains all the mineral ingredients necessary for the development of the infant; indeed, with the single exception of iron, they are present in the precise amounts in which they are needed. In this omission, however, nature is guilty of no oversight, since the infant has already been provided by the time of birth with a rich supply of iron.

THE TECHNIQUE OF NURSING.--Since the mother should have opportunity to recuperate from the fatigue of labor, physicians generally recommend that an interval of at least twelve hours elapse between the birth of the infant and the time it is first put to the breast. Moreover, the best interests of the infant demand that it be kept warm and left undisturbed while becoming accustomed to its new environment. There is no immediate need of food;

and if there were, nature does not fit the mother to supply it, for at this time the breasts contain merely small quantities of colostrum.

Some babies nurse vigorously at the outset, but later, discouraged because they get so little, become indifferent and restless, or even decline to take the breast. And the mother, who is handicapped by inexperience and by the awkwardness of nursing in a recumbent position, often feels desperate. Fortunately technical difficulties are confined to the first few days, and, trying as they sometimes are, no one should be discouraged or imagine that she is incapable of nursing; for practically every woman who persists will succeed.

For a week or ten days the mother will nurse in the recumbent posture. She turns to one side or the other, according as the right or left breast is used, and holds the corresponding arm to receive and support the baby, which will lie beside her. Then with the opposite hand she holds the breast, placing her thumb above and her fingers below so as to keep it from the baby's face, for only in this way can the infant breathe freely. One must also remember that the infant draws the milk into the terminal ducts chiefly with the back of its mouth, and drains the ducts by compressing the base of the nipple with its jaws; the infant therefore should take into its mouth not only the nipple, but also the areola, the area of deeply colored skin round about it. Mothers frequently disregard these directions, and the failure of their infants to nurse properly may be thus explained, for it is impossible to secure undisturbed nursing unless they are obeyed.

Generally the breasts are employed alternately, but both may be used at each nursing if one is insufficient. To fix the duration of the nursings arbitrarily is impossible; from ten to fifteen minutes generally proves satisfactory, but in each case systematic observations of the change in the baby's weight, of the character of its stools, and of its general condition must determine how long to leave it at the breast. The common error, unfortunately, is to be over-indulgent, and, as a result, infants are more frequently ill because the nursings are too long, than too short. Furthermore, the duration of the feedings can never be gauged accurately if the infant is allowed to nap while nursing.

The successful training of a baby begins with the development of regular habits of nursing. The old-fashioned custom of allowing the baby to nurse whenever it cried, tacitly--and incorrectly--assumed that it could have no other sensation than hunger. As a matter of fact an infant may have pain from overfeeding. Again, it may be thirsty, or uncomfortable from the pricking of a pin, from the monotony of one position, from a soiled napkin, or from neglect of many simple details in its care. Any of these things make a baby cry, for it has no other means by which it can express disapproval.

So long as the breasts contain colostrum the nursings should be at least three hours apart during the day; at night it is preferable not to disturb the mother at all. As soon as milk appears the interval is usually shortened to two hours during the day. In many cases, however, the three-hour interval will be retained even after the milk appears, for otherwise the infant may not become hungry and will fail to nurse as strongly as it should. The following schedule is adapted to the average infant:

Age Interval During Total Number the Day of Feedings From 1st to 4th week 2 hours 9 " 4th " 8th " 2-1/2 " 8 " 2nd " 4th month 3 " 7 " 4th " 10th " 3 " 6 " 10th " 12th " 4 " 5

After the first few days most young infants require one feeding in the middle of the night, which is usually given about 2 A.M. The day feedings then begin at 6 A.M., and are repeated at regular intervals until 9 or 10 P.M. The daily bath should be scheduled so that a feeding will be due just after the bath has been completed. If asleep when the next succeeding feeding falls due, the infant should not be waked, but at other times nothing should interfere with the regularity of the schedule. Occasionally there may be difficulty in getting the child to nurse during the day, but it must be taught to do so; otherwise it will want to nurse throughout the night.

At no time should an infant remain in the bed with its mother after it has finished nursing; at night this rule must be rigidly enforced, for mothers have been known to fall asleep and smother the baby, an accident known as over-lying. Infants can frequently be trained to go without feeding in the middle of the night even when a month old; and such training is always advisable, since it affords the mother opportunity for six or eight hours' continuous sleep.

Before and after each nursing the mothers' nipple should be cleansed with a solution of boric acid made by placing a tablespoonful of the powder in a tumbler which is then filled with water. Such cleansing protects the breasts against infection, a complication which the nursing mother must spare no pains to prevent. Now and then, in spite of conscientious efforts to harden them, the nipples become sore. If they crack, the baby's mouth must not come in direct contact with them, since nursing with a cracked nipple is a common source of a gathered breast. Fortunately when a nipple cracks we may employ a shield, obtainable at any drug-store, which enables the infant to nurse without any danger to the mother. Most babies will take the shield as well as the breast itself; nevertheless, its use should be discontinued as soon as the nipple heals, for while the shield is used the secretion of milk is not stimulated as vigorously as when the infant nurses directly from the breast. In the rare cases in which the shield cannot be used satisfactorily the infant must be taken from the breast temporarily and given a bottle. Radical as this advice may appear, the mother must consent to follow it, for, as I have pointed out, to permit an infant to nurse a cracked nipple is extremely hazardous. When treatment is begun promptly the cracks will generally heal within twenty-four hours.

HYGIENE OF THE MOTHER.--Since the mammary glands manufacture their product from the constituents of the mother's blood and their activity is controlled by her nerves, it is clear that her physical condition and her state of mind will influence the secretion of milk. Intelligent women who understand this desire to know how they should live that they may best insure an ample supply of good milk. Fortunately the first important step toward success has been taken when a mother wishes to nurse her baby; but there are also necessary wholesome food, habits conducive to health, and a mind free from worry.

It is unfortunate that current beliefs throw many restrictions about nursing-mothers which are unreasonable and unsupported by scientific investigation. There was a time when mothers did not question their ability to nurse, they assumed this duty as a matter of course. Indeed, they were compelled to do so, since refined methods of artificial feeding had not as yet been devised. Among the agricultural class, even to-day, it is exceptional for mothers to fail to nurse their children, if they are provided with the ordinary comforts of life. But women who live at the higher tension of city life are frequently unsuccessful, because they are more inclined to be nervous or because they disregard, among other things, the need of fresh air, plain food, or regular habits. It is wrong to suppose that elaborate rules of conduct are necessary for nursing mothers; the instruction they require is simple and scarcely different from that to be given anyone who desires good health. If she lead a wholesome existence a woman will not only nurse her child successfully but will gain in strength.

Diet.--In manufacturing centers, where a large proportion of the women are employed in confining work, the percentage of mothers who are able to nurse their children is exceedingly small; consequently the infant mortality is very high. Better nourishment for the mother, it has seemed, would render her more capable of successful lactation, and would decrease or even eliminate badly executed artificial feeding, and would therefore reduce the death rate among the babies. In a few foreign cities the idea has been put into practice. Free restaurants have been established for working mothers, and they have thus been enabled to perform their maternal duties much more successfully. Incidentally it has been shown that nourishment may be supplied mother and infant at a smaller cost than proper artificial food for the infant alone.

The quantity of nourishment required by nursing mothers is not so large as might be expected, and in many instances it is over-feeding rather than under-feeding that must be guarded against. Very accurate observations have been made which indicate that during the early weeks of nursing no more food is needed than at other times; in all probability this remains true throughout the whole period of lactation. Over-eating, as many of us know, is a frequent cause of indigestion. It is of the first importance, therefore, that nursing mothers should not take more food than they can assimilate, for indigestion will provoke disturbances in the milk which in turn will make the baby uncomfortable. For a similar reason mothers should have their meals at regular intervals.

As a rule the appetite is a reliable guide not only as to how much to eat, but also as to the choice of food, for without exception what is good for the mother is good also for the child. Generally the diet should be a mixed one, consisting of milk, gruels, soups, vegetables, bread, and meat. In order that monotony may not dull the appetite, no one article of food should be employed continuously. With this exception food should be selected with regard only for its wholesomeness and digestibility. All food is milk-making food; no sharp distinctions between the various kinds can be recognized. Milk, because it contains all the elements necessary for perfect nutrition, is particularly wholesome. Water also, since it forms such a large proportion of their milk, should be taken freely by nursing mothers. Generally it proves advantageous to take milk or some other nutritious drink between meals and again before retiring at night, but the danger of ruining in this way the appetite for solid food must not be overlooked.

It ought to be unnecessary to say that a nursing mother should deny herself any article of food, no matter how much she may want it, if she knows it will disagree with her; but she must remember also that the same article of food will not necessarily disagree with other mothers. Generalizations of this kind are largely responsible for the wrongful tendency to reject from the dietary many altogether harmless articles. There would be little left for a nursing mother to eat if she avoided every article of food which one person or another assures her will damage her milk.

No belief regarding what a nursing mother should eat is held more widely, I suppose, than that she should abstain from salads, tomatoes, and fruits which contain acid. This view is erroneous. The very idea upon which it is based is incorrect, since acids are neutralized as soon as they pass from the stomach to the intestines and cannot enter the milk. With certain persons some varieties of fruit invariably cause indigestion. Lactation does not correct such an individual peculiarity, and a nursing mother who knows she possesses it will act accordingly. Occasionally those who have no such idiosyncrasy worry after they have eaten something which contains an acid because they have heard it will do harm. In such cases it is the mental state of the woman which disturbs her milk and upsets the baby. With the exception of those who have such an idiosyncrasy and those inclined to worry, nursing mothers may partake of fruits and salads with impunity.

There are vegetables, of which the onion and turnip are good examples, that contain ingredients that find their way unaltered into the milk. So long as these do not disturb the mother their presence has no unfavorable influence upon the child. Similarly a number of substances appear in the milk when administered as medicine to the mother. In one way this is fortunate, for under certain circumstances it provides a very satisfactory method of treating unhealthy children without giving the medicine directly. In another respect, however, it is a disadvantage, for it sometimes interferes with giving the mother purgatives, which she may need. So far as possible, therefore, the taking of medicine should be limited during lactation, and certainly no drug should be employed without the advice of a physician.

Time and again some drug, some beverage, usually one that contains alcohol, or some special article of food has been recommended as a means of increasing an inadequate secretion of milk, but thus far all attempts in this direction have failed of general application. There are at present on the market widely advertised preparations for which astounding efficiency is claimed. None of them, however, has a definite or consistent value; and it is unfortunately true that no substance has yet been discovered that has the specific action of increasing the production of milk.

Psychic Influence.--Although the nerves of the breast which regulate the secretion of milk do their work whether the mother wills it or not, her state of mind has an influence over the process, just as it has over digestion. No one doubts that our minds influence our digestions as has been so clearly proved by the skillful experiments of Pawlow, an eminent Russian physiologist. Cheerfulness promotes perfect assimilation of the food, whereas mental depression decreases the secretion of the digestive juices or checks them altogether. In a similar way, perhaps, we shall some day have explained to us the unquestioned fact that mothers who maintain a happy disposition nurse their babies efficiently, while those who are inclined to worry often experience real or imaginary troubles with lactation.

The most striking manifestations of such psychic influences are those in which, as a result of some strong passion or deep sorrow, the secretion of milk suddenly ceases altogether. Fortunately such effects occur rarely and are never permanent. After a few hours at most the secretion is reestablished; and if there are alterations in the quality of the milk, these will correct themselves just as quickly.

More common, and therefore much more important, are cases in which, because the mother allows herself day after day to worry over one thing or another, the secretion of milk suffers permanent disturbance in quantity or in quality. Sometimes worrying lest the milk will be unsatisfactory causes it to become so. Generally, however, unnecessary anxiety for the baby is to blame.

Again and again, when there is really nothing out of the way, inexperienced mothers make themselves miserable because they fear something may go wrong. Such a state of mind always invites trouble; not infrequently it is the direct cause of insufficient or unwholesome milk. The self-assurance gained through taking care of the first baby is responsible more than anything else for the greater success mothers have in nursing subsequent children.

The mother who is nursing her first baby should take success for granted, and never mistrust her ability to succeed. If the physician has been asked to visit the baby regularly, as was suggested at the beginning of this chapter, he will quickly detect the evidence of failure should failure be imminent. His opinions should be accepted and his directions followed, for by so doing the mother will most readily acquire the assurance which is so necessary to success. The habit, easily fallen into, of paying attention to promiscuous advice is unwholesome, for such advice is injudiciously given and is usually incorrect. More often than not the counsel of well-meaning friends only serves to perplex and distress the mother.

Recreation and Rest.--Next to worry no influence upon lactation is more detrimental than neglect of recreation and rest. Both are very necessary to a nursing mother, for without them she will soon begin to exaggerate minor troubles and even to worry though nothing is wrong. A mother who has the care of a baby added to other responsibilities may have extraordinary difficulty in finding time for outdoor exercise, for congenial companionship, or for diversion of any kind. Occasionally it may seem almost impossible even to get time for sleep, a necessity so fundamental to health that, as we should expect, a mother deprived of it would fail utterly in nursing her infant. Difficult as it may seem, however, the mother must find time for recreation, for if she does not there will follow disturbances, generally in the quantity, or sometimes in the quality, of her milk.

Keeping in mind that whatever benefits the mother will react favorably upon the infant, one should regulate exercise during lactation with regard to the kind and the amount of exercise to which she has been previously accustomed. Walking usually fulfils all the requirements satisfactorily, and there is ordinarily no reason why nursing mothers should not participate in sports that are unattended by violent exertion. Exhausting sports, however, must be shunned, because fatigue has the same injurious effect upon the secretion of milk as lack of exercise.

As might be expected, women who are frail are most susceptible to the strain of nursing, especially if they fail to get sufficient rest. All nursing mothers ought to have at least eight hours of sleep in the twenty-four. The night-feeding, generally advisable for the first six to eight weeks, does not break the mother's rest longer than half an hour if the baby is well trained. But if a baby that has not been properly trained turns night into day and keeps the mother awake for long intervals, the milk will quickly deteriorate. Under such circumstances someone must relieve the mother of the care of the infant during the night; she should not be disturbed even to nurse it. The night-feeding will then be supplied artificially; as will also one feeding during the day in order that the mother may have opportunity for exercise and diversion.

THE SUPPLEMENTARY BOTTLE.--At first glance it may seem that in the suggestion that the infant be given one artificial feeding each day the mother's comfort alone has been considered. As a matter of fact, however, the adoption of the plan benefits mother and infant alike. The diversion and recreation which the mother, thus relieved of her maternal duties for from four to six hours, has time to secure becomes a direct benefit to the infant. Not infrequently by pursuing this plan, mothers who would otherwise be incapable of nursing are assured successful lactation. The child, moreover, having thus become accustomed to the bottle, is much more easily denied the breast when the time for weaning comes.

Objections have been raised to giving the baby even one bottle when the mother has an ample supply of milk, but none of them are valid. Since cow's milk is acknowledged to be less easy of digestion than is human milk, it will occur to someone that there is danger of upsetting the baby by giving it a bottle. But this need not be feared; extensive experience has shown that if an infant is getting human milk of satisfactory quality at all its feedings during the twenty-four hours, save one or two, at these times it will digest properly modified cow's milk without the least inconvenience. Nor is it true that if once a day cow's milk is substituted for that of the mother, the infant will come to prefer the bottle to the breast. There is no danger, on the other hand, that the mother's milk will dry up. Very thorough investigation of these objections has failed to substantiate them in the least.

Of course, it will be necessary in preparing the supplementary feeding to take the same precautions as if the infant were on the bottle exclusively. To avoid contamination of the milk care must be exercised to have everything perfectly clean that comes in contact with it. And it will be necessary also to vary from time to time both the strength and the amount of the feeding. These alterations will be made most successfully if left to the judgment of a physician who is familiar with the development of the infant and who may be guided accordingly.

WEANING.--Occasionally, even before they are delivered, women express the conviction that they will be incapable of nursing. A few mothers who take this attitude, which it would seem is becoming more and more common, make no attempt at nursing, and others give it up after a very short trial. Premature weaning is practiced among the women of two widely different classes: those who are unwilling to deny themselves social pleasures, and those who, because they must earn a living, cannot be encumbered with maternal duties. A still larger class, however, are those mothers who wean the baby for neither of these reasons, but rather because they become discouraged and conclude that there is something wrong with their milk. In this way many infants are weaned without sufficient reason. Before giving up nursing her child a mother should submit several samples of the milk for analysis. If it is unfit for the infant, reliable evidence of the fact will often be secured in this way.

With the exception of tuberculosis, physicians recognize no condition that necessarily unfits a mother for nursing. As we have already seen, pregnancy is generally incompatible with lactation; in the event of conception the mother's milk almost always takes on qualities which render it unsatisfactory for the infant, and yet occasionally pregnancy advances several months before these changes in the milk occur. Meanwhile the infant suffers no inconvenience, and often in these cases the symptoms of threatened miscarriage give the first intimation of the mother's condition. Under all circumstances, however, nursing should cease as soon as the mother recognizes that she is pregnant, for probably no woman is strong enough to provide nourishment for her infant and for the development of the embryo simultaneously.

Menstruation, on the other hand, rarely if ever provides a good and sufficient reason for weaning. In the great majority of instances this function is re-established before lactation ends. There may be a reduction in the amount of milk during menstruation, but if the infant has been given the breast as usual, the supply increases as soon as the period ends. Qualitative disturbances which would render the milk unfit for use are practically never a consequence of menstruation.

It may happen as the infant grows older that the flow of milk will diminish; then the breast feedings will of necessity be more frequently replaced by the bottle, and the question of weaning will settle itself. But if the time of weaning is a matter of choice, it should be approximately coincident with certain notable developments in the infant's digestive functions, which occur toward the end of the first year. The fact that the infant is prepared to take other food is outwardly shown by the appearance of teeth, of which there are usually six or eight at the end of the year.

If the suggestion regarding the daily substitution of one bottle for the mother's milk has been adopted, there will be no difficulty in discontinuing breast-feeding whenever it is desirable; otherwise an infant may raise strong objection to the change. The mother, on the other hand, will not be seriously inconvenienced by the weaning, provided she leaves her breasts alone.

Until recently mothers were advised to employ a very elaborate treatment for drying up the breasts. The diet was restricted, and as far as possible liquids of every kind were forbidden; strong purgatives were administered daily; and, in addition, the breasts were covered with some ointment, swathed in cotton, and tightly compressed with a bandage. Fortunately, we now realize that none of these measures are required. When nursing is discontinued the breasts are apt to become distended and uncomfortable. They require support while the distention lasts, which is never very long, and if they become painful, medicine may be employed to give relief. But other measures, some of which occasionally do harm, are absolutely unnecessary, for, at whatever period of lactation the breasts cease to be used, they dry up spontaneously.

GLOSSARY

[Footnote: The Century Dictionary has been freely used for these definitions.]

ABNORMAL.--Irregular; deviating from the natural or standard type.

ABORTIFACIENT.--Whatever is used to produce an abortion.

ABORTION.--The expulsion of the embryo during the first four months of pregnancy.

AFTER-BIRTH.--The mass of tissue expelled from the uterus at the end of labor. It includes the placenta, the umbilical cord, and the membranes of the ovum.

ALIMENTARY CANAL.--The digestive tract. It begins with the mouth, includes the stomach and the intestines, and ends with the rectum.

AMNIOTIC FLUID.--The liquid inclosed within the amniotic membrane.

AMNIOTIC MEMBRANE.--The innermost of the two membranes which envelop the embryo; the lining membrane of the closed sac familiarly called "the bag of waters."

ANEMIA.--A deficiency of some of the constituents of the blood.

ANATOMY.--The science which deals with the structure of the body.

ANTISEPTIC.--Anything which destroys bacteria.

AREOLA.--The colored, circular area about the nipple.

ARTERY.--A vessel through which the blood flows away from the heart.

ASEPSIS.--The exclusion of disease-producing bacteria.

ASEPTIC.--Free from injurious bacteria.

ASPHYXIA.--The extreme condition caused by lack of oxygen in the blood, brought about by interrupted breathing.

ASSIMILATION.--The process by which living creatures digest and absorb nutriment so that it becomes part of the substance composing them.

ATROPHY.--To waste away.

AUTO-INTOXICATION.--Poisoning by material formed within one's body.

BACTERIA (the plural of bacterium).--Exceedingly minute, spherical, oblong, or cylindrical cells which are concerned in putrefactive processes. Some varieties cause disease.

BACTERIAL DECOMPOSITION.--Putrefaction brought about by the action of bacteria.

BIOLOGY.--The science which deals with the phenomena of life.

BIRTH-CANAL.--The passage through which the child enters the world. It is composed of the uterus and the vagina, and is surrounded by the pelvic bones.

BLADDER.--A thin, distensible sack acting as a reservoir for the urine between the time it is secreted by the kidneys and leaves the body.

BREECH.--The buttocks.

CESAREAN OPERATION.--The operation by which the child is taken out of the uterus by an incision through the abdominal wall.

CALORIE.--The unit ordinarily employed by scientists to measure heat.

CAPILLARIES.--The minute blood vessels which form a network between the terminations of the arteries and the beginnings of the veins.

CARBOHYDRATE.--Any one of a group of chemical substances of which starch and sugar are the most familiar members.

CARBONIC ACID GAS.--An animal waste product eliminated in the breath. In daylight plants absorb it energetically from the atmosphere through their leaves, and decompose it, assimilating the carbon, and returning the oxygen to the air.

CARTILAGE.--A firm, elastic tissue; gristle. From this material many of the bones develop.

CATHETERIZE.--To empty the bladder by means of a tube-like instrument which is introduced into the passage through which the urine normally leaves the bladder.

CELL.--One of the microscopical structural units which make up our bodies.

CELL-DIVISION.--The process by which a single cell becomes two cells.

CEREBRUM.--The portion of the brain which is the seat of mental activity.

CHORIONIC MEMBRANE.--The outermost of the two membranes which surround the embryo.

CHROMATIN.--A substance within the nucleus of a cell which has a special affinity for certain staining agents.

CHROMOSOMES.--One of the pieces into which the chromatin is broken during the act of cell-division.

CLINICAL.--Pertaining to the sick-bed.

COLOSTRUM.--The fluid secreted by the breasts during pregnancy and for two or three days after the birth of the child.

CONTRACTION.--The act by which the muscle fibers of the uterus become shorter and press upon its contents.

CURETTAGE.--Scraping out the lining of the uterus.

DELIVERY.--The birth of the child.

DIAGNOSIS.--The determination of either normal or abnormal states of the body.

DIAPHRAGM.--The muscular partition between the chest and the abdomen.

DIETETIC.--Pertaining to the diet.

DUCT.--A tube which conveys the secretion from a gland.

EMBRYO.--The offspring before it has assumed the distinctive form and structure of the parent.

ENEMA.--A quantity of fluid injected into the rectum.

ENGAGEMENT.--The entrance of the fetus into the birth-canal.

ETHNOLOGY.--The science which deals with the character, customs, and institutions of races of men.

EUGENICS.--The science which deals with the improvement of the human race by better breeding. (Davenport.)

EXCRETION.--Waste substance thrown off from the body.

FEBRILE.--Attended with fever.

FETUS.--The unborn child after the third month of development.

FOOD-STUFF.--Anything used for the sustenance of man.

FUNCTION.--The discharge of its duty by any organ of the body.

GASTRIC JUICE.--The digestive fluid secreted by the wall of the stomach.

GERMINAL CELLS.--The structural units from which a new individual takes origin. The cell contributed by the mother is called an egg- cell or ovum; that contributed by the father, a spermatozoon.

GESTATION.--Same as pregnancy.

GLAND.--An organ which separates certain substances from the blood, and pours out a material, usually fluid, peculiar to itself.

HYGIENE.--That department of medical knowledge which relates to the preservation of health; sanitary science.

INANITION.--The condition which results from insufficient nourishment.

INFECTION.--A disease due to bacteria.

INTESTINE.--The bowels; the long membranous tube extending from the stomach to the rectum.

INVOLUTION.--The process by which the uterus returns after child-birth to its former size and position.

LACTATION.--The secretion of milk.

LIGAMENT.--A band of tissue serving to bind one part of the body to another.

LIGATURE.--Anything that serves for tying a blood-vessel.

LOCHIA.--The discharge continuing for several weeks after the birth of a child.

LOTION.--Any liquid holding in solution medicinal substances intended for application to the skin.

LUNAR MONTH.--A month of twenty-eight days.

MAMMAL.--The highest order of animal, namely, one which suckles its young.

MAMMARY.--Relating to the breast.

MASTICATION.--The act of chewing.

MENOPAUSE.--The permanent abolishment of the menstrual process, which generally occurs between the 45th and the 50th years.

MICRO-ORGANISMS.--Bacteria and other living agents of disease which are visible only with the aid of the microscope.

MISCARRIAGE.--The termination of pregnancy prior to the seventh month.

MUCOUS MEMBRANE.--The lining of certain cavities of the body, such as the mouth, stomach, intestine, uterus, etc.

MUCUS.--The material manufactured by the glands in a mucous membrane.

MUSCLE-FIBERS.--The muscle-cells.

NARCOTICS.--Drugs which produce sleep.

NITROGEN.--One of the chemical elements.

NUCLEUS.--A clearly defined area found in every cell which seems to be its seat of government.

OBSTETRICS.--The branch of medicine which deals with the treatment and care of women during pregnancy and child-birth.

OVARY.--The organ which contains the egg-cells or ova.

OVIDUCTS.--Two tubes, each of which leads from the neighborhood of one of the ovaries; both terminate in the uterus.

OVUM.--An egg: the cell contributed by the mother to her offspring.

OXYGEN.--One of the chemical elements.

PATHOLOGY.--The branch of medicine which deals with the altered structure and activity of diseased organs.

PEPSIN.--A ferment found in the digestive juice secreted by the stomach.

PELVIC FLOOR.--The muscles, ligaments, and other tissues which form the bottom of the basin inclosed between the hips.

PELVIS.--The bony ring formed chiefly by the hip bones. Posteriorly the ring is completed by the sacrum.

PERINEUM.--The region extending backward from the outlet of the vagina to the rectum; it is the most essential part of the pelvic floor.

PHYSIOLOGY.--Scientific knowledge of the manner in which the various parts of the body perform their duties.

PIGMENT.--Any coloring matter.

PLACENTA.--The organ through which the communication between the mother and the offspring is established. One of its surfaces is attached to the wall of the uterus; at about the middle point of the other surface the umbilical cord takes its origin.

PRENATAL.--Pertaining to the period before birth.

PROTEIN.--A food-stuff which is distinguished by the fact that it contains nitrogen and is a tissue builder.

PROTOPLASM.--The living substance in the cells which compose our bodies.

PUBERTY.--Sexual maturity in human beings.

PUBIC BONES.--The part of the pelvis which forms an arch in front of the bladder.

PUERPERIUM.--The same as the lying-in period.

RETINA.--The innermost coat of the eye-ball and the one which receives visual impressions.

RICKETS.--A disease of infancy characterized by softening of the bones.

SECRETION.--The product of the activity of a gland.

SEDIMENT.--The material which settles to the bottom of any liquid.

SPERMATOZOON (plural spermatozoa).--The microscopic cell contributed by the male parent, which stimulates the ovum to begin its development.

SUPPOSITORY.--A medicinal substance made into the form of a cone to be introduced into the rectum.

TERM.--The time of expected delivery.

THERAPEUTIC.--Concerned with the treatment of disease.

THYMUS GLAND.--A structure located behind the breast bone near the root of the neck. Only traces of it are found in adult life.

TISSUE.--An aggregation of similar cells in a definite fabric, as muscle, nerve, gland, etc.

TUBES.--The oviducts.

UMBILICAL CORD.--The structure carrying the blood vessels which pass between the placenta and the child's navel.

UTERUS.--The womb: a hollow muscular organ designed to receive, protect, nourish, and expel the product of conception.

VAGINA.--The canal through which the child passes from the uterus into the world.

VEIN.--A vessel through which the blood flows back to the heart.

VERNIX.--The fatty substance deposited over the skin of the newly born infant.

VIABLE.--Capable of living.

VILLI (singular villus).--The microscopic, finger-like processes which hang from one of the surfaces of the placenta and are surrounded by the mother's blood.

VISCERA.--The internal organs which occupy the cavities of the chest and the abdomen.

VULVA.--The folds of tissue which surround the outlet of the vagina.

www.ingramcontent.com/pod-product-compliance
Lightning Source LLC
Chambersburg PA
CBHW070856180526
45168CB00005B/1844

* 9 7 8 1 5 1 1 9 9 0 7 6 9 *